Manual of Artificial Cardiac Pacing

Manual of Artificial Cardiac Pacing

by

Edward K. Chung, M.D., F.A.C.P., F.A.C.C.

Professor of Medicine
Jefferson Medical College of
Thomas Jefferson University
and
Director of the Heart Station and
Attending Physician (Cardiologist)
Thomas Jefferson University Hospital
Philadelphia, Pennsylvania

UNIVERSITY PARK PRESS • Baltimore

University Park Press
International Publishers in Medicine and Human Services
300 North Charles Street
Baltimore, Maryland 21201

Typeset by Waldman Graphics, Inc.

Manufactured in the United States of America by Kingsport Press

Library of Congress Cataloging in Publication Data

Chung, Edward K.
Manual of artificial cardiac pacing.
Bibliography: p.
Includes index.
1. Pacemaker, Artificial (Heart) I. Title.
[DNLM: 1. Arrhythmia—Handbooks. 2. Cardiac pacing, Artificial—Handbooks. 3. Pacemaker, Artificial—Handbooks. WG 168 C559m]
RC684.P3C48 1983 617'.4120645 83-6553
ISBN 0-8391-1877-5

To My Wife, Lisa and
My Children, Linda and Christopher

Contents

Preface

It has been well documented that artificial (electronic) cardiac pacing is one of the most important and reliable ways to manage various cardiac arrhythmias, particularly bradyarrhythmias. Until 5 to 10 years ago, the primary indication for permanent pacing had been in the treatment of complete A-V block. At the present time, the most common indication for permanent pacing is in the treatment of sick sinus syndrome. Hence this syndrome is discussed in great detail in this book. In addition, artificial pacing with an overdriving pacing rate is often a lifesaving measure for refractory tachyarrhythmias.

Approximately 250,000 people (500,000 people according to some reports) live with artificial cardiac pacemakers in America alone, and 25,000 to 40,000 (100,000 to 110,000 according to some medical reports) new patients annually require artificial pacemaker implantation. This means that each physician who takes care of cardiac patients must be fully familiar with all aspects of artificial pacing. Thus follow-up care of patients who have undergone artificial pacemaker implantation is discussed in detail.

The intention of this book is *not* to describe every aspect of pacing in detail. Rather, only clinically pertinent information regarding artificial pacing is discussed, so that the book is concise and practical. The format of the book is somewhat comparable to that seen in cookbooks, which can be extremely beneficial to cardiologists as well as to busy practitioners who are *not* specializing in cardiology. In addition, the book can be valuable to all medical house officers, emergency room physicians, anesthesiologists, medical students, and cardiac care nurses. Furthermore, technical personnel, sales representatives, and other individuals who are closely related to the field of artificial pacemakers may also obtain benefit by reading this Manual.

It has been my pleasure to share the work to complete this valuable Manual with the staff of University Park Press, particularly Mrs. Ruby Richardson, Senior Editor.

Edward K. Chung, M.D.

Bryn Mawr, Pennsylvania

About the Author

Edward K. Chung, M.D., F.A.C.P., F.A.C.C.

Fellow, American College of Cardiology
Former Governor for West Virginia, American College of Cardiology
Fellow, American College of Physicians
Member, American Federation for Clinical Research
Member, American Heart Association
Member, American Medical Association
Member, World Congress of Cardiology
Member, Asian Pacific Congress of Cardiology
Member, International Congress of Electrocardiology
Member, Pennsylvania Medical Society
Member, Philadelphia County Medical Society
Member, Korean Medical Association

Editorial Board Member for:
Cardiology,
The Journal of Electrocardiology,
Heart and Lung,
Primary Cardiology,
Cardiology Clinics,
and
Hospital Physician

The author and the publisher have exercised great care to ensure that the drug dosages, formulas, and other information presented in this book are accurate and in accord with the professional standards in effect at the time of publication. Readers are, however, advised to always check the manufacturer's product information sheet that is packaged with the respective products to be fully informed of changes in recommended dosages, contraindications, and the like before prescribing or administering any drug.

Introduction

1

It has been well documented that artificial (electronic) cardiac pacing is one of the most important and reliable ways to manage various cardiac arrhythmias, particularly the bradyarrhythmias. Until 5 to 10 years ago, the primary indication for permanent artificial pacing was for the treatment of complete atrioventricular (A-V) block. The most common indication of permanent artificial pacemakers at the present time, however, is in the treatment of the sick sinus syndrome (SSS). In addition, artificial pacing with an overdriving pacing rate (faster-than-usual pacing rate) is often a lifesaving measure in patients with refractory tachyarrhythmias. The term ''bradytachyarrhythmia syndrome'' is used when the abnormal heart rhythms consist of a rapid rhythm as well as a slow rhythm. In this case, artificial cardiac pacing has a very important role because drug therapy alone is usually ineffective. Bradytachyarrhythmia syndrome is usually a late manifestation of SSS (see Chapter 4).

The artificial cardiac pacemaker functions in a manner similar to that of the natural pacemaker. Electrical impulses are generated by small batteries and then travel through small wires to the heart. The artificial pacemaker is timed to produce the electrical impulses (usually about 70 to 72 beats/min) just like the cardiac impulses initiated by the natural pacemaker (sinus node). In most cases the heart is capable of pumping adequate amounts of blood under the control of an artificial pacemaker.

Approximately 250,000 people (500,000 according to some reports) live with artificial cardiac pacemakers in America alone, and 25,000 to 40,000 (100,000 to 110,000 according to some medical reports) new patients require artificial pacemaker implantation annually. Although it is difficult to know exactly how many people live with an artificial pacemaker at the present time worldwide, it is estimated to be at least 500,000 (750,000 to 1,000,000 according to some reports). The total number of artificial pacemakers sold within the last 20 years is estimated to be at least 1.5 million to 2 million, possibly more. It is clear that artificial cardiac pacing not only prolongs human lives but significantly improves the quality of life. Long-term administration of various drugs (e.g., isoproterenol, atropine, epinephrine) for bradyarrhythmias is no longer necessary because of the ready availability of artificial pacemakers in most developed countries.

The fundamental principles for the utilization of an artificial pacemaker were established as early as 1932 by Hyman and later by Callaghan and Bigelow in 1951. External cardiac pacing was introduced into clinical medicine in 1952 by Zoll. In 1957 temporary direct myocardial stimulation in the treatment of complete A-V block was introduced by Weirich et al., and the value of a transistorized, self-contained, implantable pacemaker for long-term correction of chronic complete A-V block was established in 1960 by Chardack et al. Until several years ago, mercury-zinc cells had been used for the energy source, but today a lithium battery has entirely replaced the mercury-zinc battery for all types of artificial pacemaker. A lithium battery lasts 10 to 12 years in most clinical circumstances. The earlier pacemakers lasted only 15 to 18 months, and so frequent replacement of the pulse generator was required. The nuclear-powered pacemaker was introduced to clinical medicine about 20 years ago, but it is not commonly used.

There are many types of artificial pacemaker in the market, but the most commonly used model is a demand ventricular pacemaker. The demand pacemaker has a sensing device which cuts the pacemaker off if the natural heart rhythm is faster than the preset pacing rate. When the patient's own rhythm becomes slower than the preset pacing rate, the sensing device turns the artificial pacemaker on again. In other words, the demand artificial pacemaker works only when needed. This is why the term "demand," or "standby," pacemaker is used. During the past few years, multiprogrammable pacemakers have been introduced in clinical medicine. With this new type of artificial pacemaker, various functions (e.g., pacing rate, energy output, sensitivity) of the pacemaker can easily be controlled and adjusted noninvasively after implantation, thereby providing the best pacing for a given individual. The multiprogrammable pacemakers will eventually replace all nonprogrammable pacemakers in the near future. The average cost of the artificial pacemaker ranges from $2,000 to $3,000. The total cost for implantation of an artificial pacemaker, including the surgeon's fee, hospitalization, and various laboratory tests, is about $6,000 to $7,000 in most hospitals.

After implantation of an artificial pacemaker, the patient should have periodic medical checkups and should carry out the necessary daily care. These precautions are important because the artificial pacemaker requires care like any other mechanical device, and complications or malfunctions occasionally occur.

INDICATIONS FOR ARTIFICIAL PACEMAKERS

Although the precise criteria for the use of a temporary or a permanent pacemaker vary slightly from one institution to another, the following conditions are generally accepted as requiring a pacemaker.

Short-Term Pacing (Temporary Pacing)

1. Symptomatic second degree or third degree A-V block, especially during acute myocardial infarction (MI). It should be noted that A-V block per se does not require artificial pacing.
2. Symptomatic and drug-resistant sinus arrhythmias, including sinus bradycardia, sinus arrest, sinoatrial (S-A) block, and A-V junctional bradyarrhythmias (often manifestations of SSS).
3. Bifascicular (BFB) and incomplete trifascicular (TFB) blocks associated with acute anterior MI, usually (prophylactic pacing). This is because these findings are often followed by a slow ventricular escape rhythm due to complete A-V block [infranodal A-V block or complete bilateral bundle branch block (BBBB)].
4. Emergency treatment for Adams-Stokes syndrome, symptomatic BBBB, and SSS.
5. Before or during implantation of a permanent pacemaker when the patient is symptomatic (e.g., syncope or near-syncope).
6. Prophylactic pacing during major surgery when Adams-Stokes syndrome and/or marked bradyarrhythmias are anticipated.
7. Drug-resistant tachyarrhythmias, using an overdriving pacing rate.

At present the most commonly used pacemaker for short-term pacing is the temporary transvenous type. In almost all situations, a demand unit is preferable to a fixed-rate unit. This is because normal A-V conduction may be present during the insertion of a pacemaker (especially when it is being used prophylactically) and because it is not uncommon to observe normal A-V conduction intermittently after the development of complete A-V block. A bipolar or unipolar catheter electrode is inserted via a jugular or arm vein into the right ventricle, preferably in the apical region, under direct vision utilizing fluoroscopy with an image intensifier. The blind float technique may also be used in certain cases. In this method the catheter electrode is advanced gently into position as the location of the tip is monitored by electrocardiography (ECG). The usual pacing rate is around 70 to 72 beats/min.

When physiological pacing is desired, of course, A-V sequential (bifocal) pacing mode is preferable (discussed later). One of the important beneficial effects of atrial pacing is its ability to suppress a variety of ectopic tachyarrhythmias, particularly those of supraventricular origin. Thus atrial pacing, coronary sinus pacing, and A-V sequential pacing are advantageous in the treatment of bradytachyarrhythmia syndrome or drug-resistant tachyarrhythmias. When there is significant A-V conduction disturbance under these circumstances, A-V sequential pacing (bifocal pacing) must be carried out. Indications for temporary pacing are discussed in detail in Chapter 6.

Indications for Long-Term (Permanent) Pacing

The decision as to whether long-term pacing is indicated is very serious, because if the pacemaker is implanted the patient must live with it all his or her life and must observe various necessary cautions and daily care. In addition, the pulse generator should be changed every 8 to 12 years in most cases (every 3 to 6 years in older models), depending on the model. One of the most serious problems after permanent pacemaker implantation is malfunction of the unit (see Chapter 11), which may be fatal. At times it is difficult to judge whether a permanent artificial pacemaker is definitely required; there is some controversy among physicians concerning certain clinical circumstances. In general, however, long-term pacing is considered to be indicated in the following situations:

1. Symptomatic and/or advanced SSS
2. Symptomatic, chronic, second degree (usually Mobitz type II) or third degree (infranodal) A-V block
3. Complete A-V block in acute MI (regardless of the location of the MI) that lasts more than 2 to 3 weeks
4. Congenital complete A-V block
5. Symptomatic bilateral bundle branch block
6. Recurrent Adams-Stokes syndrome (usually due to Mobitz type II, advanced, or complete A-V block and SSS)
7. Recurrent drug-resistant tachyarrhythmias benefited by temporary pacing
8. Carotid sinus syncope (may or may not be due to SSS)

When the indication of a permanent pacemaker has been diagnosed, the type of pacemaker suitable for the specific patient must be determined taking into consideration the patient's age, general condition, and underlying disease. When physiological pacing is desired, A-V sequential (bifocal) pacing is preferable because the artificial pacing can provide hemodynamic consequences that are almost identical to the natural sinus rhythm, so that maximal cardiac output can be maintained. This is the reason bifocal pacing has become the most commonly used method of artificial pacing in most clinical circumstances today. One of the major advantages of atrial pacing is its ability to suppress various ectopic tachyarrhythmias, particularly those of supraventricular origin. Drug-resistant tachyarrhythmias or bradytachyarrhythmias are often best treated with atrial pacing, coronary sinus pacing, or A-V sequential pacing. Of course, the A-V sequential pacing must be used when there is significant A-V conduction disturbance under these circumstances. The fixed-rate ventricular pacemaker is seldom used in the United States today because of its frequent complications. These pacemakers are manufactured primarily for use in other countries. Ordinary demand ventricular pacing is adequate in the treatment of complete A-V block when physiological artificial pacing is considered to be *not* essential. Indications for permanent pacing are discussed in detail in Chapter 8.

Artificial Pacemakers in Acute MI

There is a significant controversy among physicians regarding the use of artificial pacemakers in patients with MI. The indications for artificial pacing vary markedly depending on the site of the MI. By and large, artificial pacing is used more frequently in patients with acute anterior MI than in those with acute diaphragmatic MI. Prophylactic artificial pacing is often indicated in acute anterior MI because one or more fascicles of the His-Purkinje network are frequently damaged. Indications for artificial pacing in MI are described in detail in Chapter 7.

TYPES OF ARTIFICIAL PACEMAKER

Fixed-Rate Ventricular Pacemakers

1. The fixed-rate pacemaker is designed to function regardless of the patient's own natural rhythm (Figure 1-1).

2. A fixed-rate ventricular pacemaker can be used with relative safety in patients with established chronic complete A-V block in whom normal A-V conduction is unlikely to occur, even temporarily.

3. In addition, older patients with relatively good cardiac function using a fixed-rate pacemaker are able to carry out their ordinary activities quite adequately because maximum cardiac output is not important for sustaining their limited physical requirements.

4. In approximately 25% of patients who require permanent pacing for Adams-Stokes syndrome, normal A-V conduction (either normal sinus rhythm or second degree A-V block) may return either temporarily or even for long periods of time. In this case, the patient's own rhythm competes with the pacemaker rhythm so that the patient may develop ventricular fibrillation (VF) as a result of the R-on-T phenomenon [where a premature ventricular (QRS) complex in the ECG interrupts the T wave of the preceding beat]. Primarily because of this, a demand pacemaker is preferable in many patients in whom normal A-V conduction may return even momentarily.

5. A fixed-rate pacemaker is often used when overdriving pacing is indicated for treatment of drug-resistant ectopic tachyarrhythmias.

6. A fixed-rate pacemaker is seldom used today because other, newer pacemakers have various superior aspects.

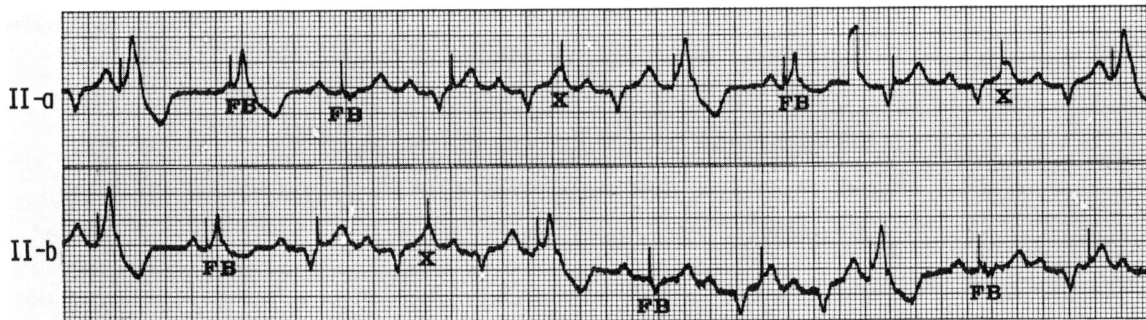

FIGURE 1-1. Leads II-a and II-b are not continuous. The basic rhythm is a sinus rhythm with first degree A-V block (P-R interval: 0.22 sec) and a fixed-rate ventricular pacemaker rhythm. Note that the pacemaker rhythm competes with the basic sinus rhythm and that there are frequent ventricular fusion beats (*FB*). The R-on-T phenomenon is observed in several areas (*X*).

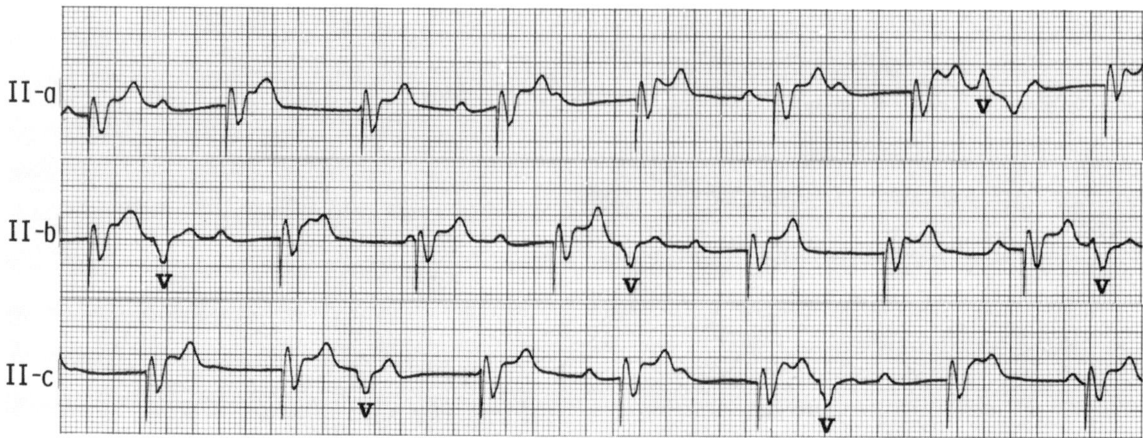

FIGURE 1-2. Leads II-a, II-b, and II-c are not continuous. The rhythm is a sinus rhythm with a demand ventricular pacemaker rhythm and frequent VPCs (*V*).

Demand (Standby) Ventricular Pacemakers

1. During the past 10 to 15 years, demand pacemakers have gradually replaced fixed-rate pacemakers because of their definite superiority. Thus competition between the natural rhythm and the artificial pacemaker rhythm can be avoided.

2. The demand ventricular pacemaker functions only when the R-R intervals of the natural rhythm exceed a preset limit (Figure 1-2). Therefore a demand pacemaker is particularly ideal for temporary pacing when bradyarrhythmias are transient or intermittent.

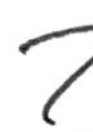

3. It is important to recognize "hysteresis" (where the interval from the natural beat to the immediately following paced beat is longer than the consecutively occurring pacing interval) in some models of demand units (Figure 1-3). Otherwise, the finding may be misdiagnosed as malfunction.

4. There are some disadvantages in using transvenous catheter electrodes, including perforation of the ventricles, failure of pacing due to migration or exit block, infection, and fracture.

Atrial-Synchronized Pacemakers

1. A more physiological type of artificial pacemaker is the atrial-synchronized pacemaker.

2. In this type of pacemaker, the pulse generator is triggered by the natural P wave of atrial depolarization, and ventricular stimulation follows after an optimal delay corresponding to the P-R interval (Figure 1-4). In other words, an atrial-synchronized pacemaker functions as an electronic bundle of His.

3. The major advantage of this type of pacemaker is its ability to provide maximum augmentation of the cardiac output at changing atrial rates in order to meet varying physiological requirements.

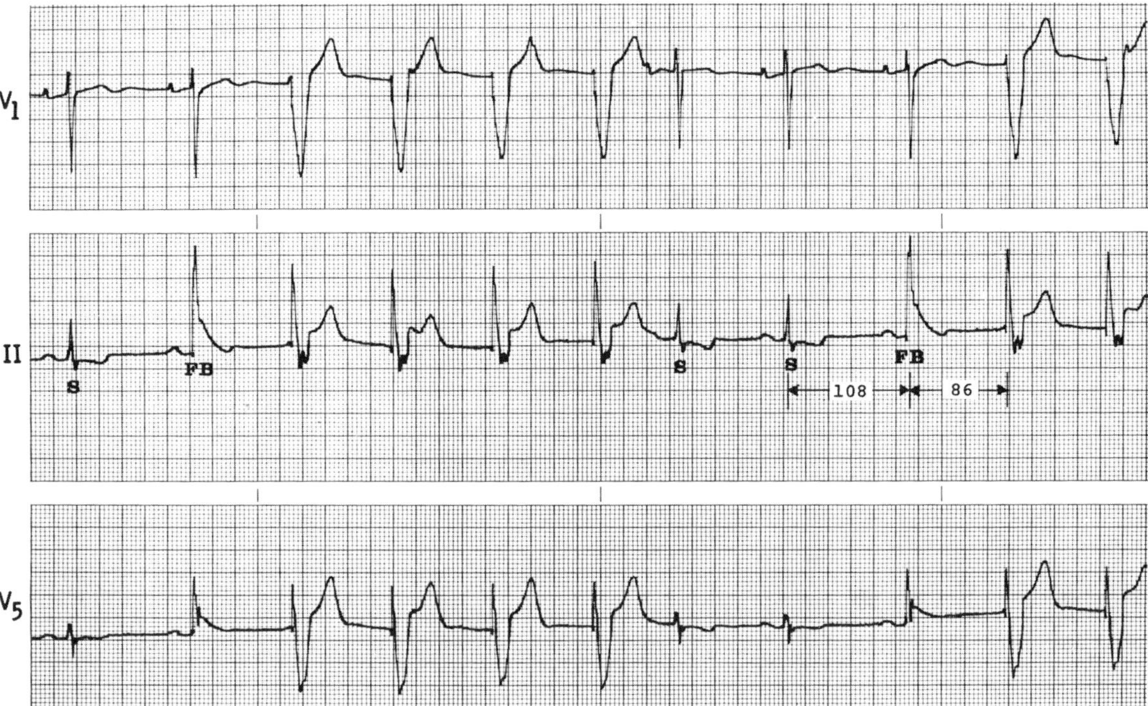

FIGURE 1-3. Leads V_1, II, and V_5 were taken simultaneously by using a three-channel recorder. The tracing shows a ventricular demand pacemaker (Medtronic model 5943) induced ventricular rhythm (rate: 67 beats/min) with intermittent sinus beats (*S*). Note that the pacemaker escape interval (1.08 sec) is much longer than the consecutively occurring pacing intervals (0.86 sec) because of hysteresis. There are occasional ventricular fusion beats (*FB*). (The numbers in this figure represent hundredths of a second.)

4. Another benefit is its utilization of the atrial contribution to ventricular filling to further augment cardiac output.

5. Thus the atrial-synchronized pacemaker becomes extremely valuable in young or active patients.

6. When atrial tachycardia or flutter occurs, the pacemaker induces A-V block of varying degree so that an optimum ventricular rate is maintained.

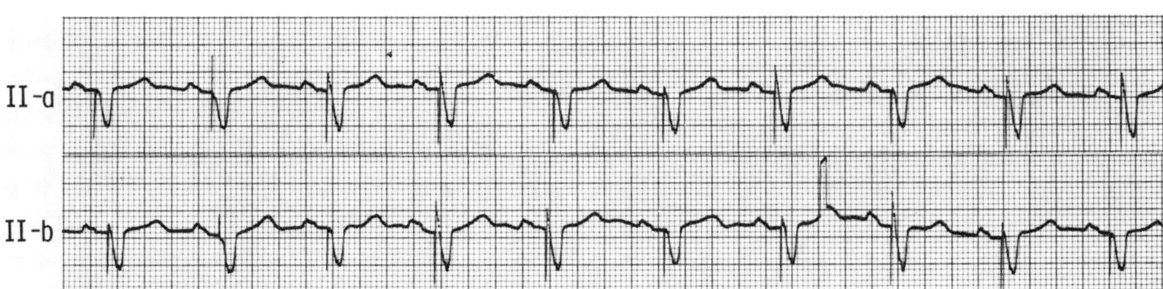

FIGURE 1-4. Leads II-a and II-b are not continuous. The rhythm is an atrial-synchronized pacemaker rhythm.

7. Although the advantages of an atrial-synchronized pacemaker are definitely known, electronic failure is frequent, and thoracotomy takes longer because of the complexity of the device.

8. An atrial-synchronized pacemaker is contraindicated in atrial fibrillation (AF), marked sinus bradycardia, unstable atrial activity (e.g., S-A block), sinus arrest, and atrial standstill.

Bifocal (A-V Sequential) Demand Pacemakers

1. The bifocal (A-V sequential) demand pacemaker consists of two demand units, a conventional QRS-inhibited ventricular pacemaker, and a QRS-inhibited atrial pacemaker (Figure 1-5).

2. In this model the escape interval of the atrial pacemaker is designed to be shorter than that of the ventricular pacemaker. Thus the difference between these two escape intervals is a determining factor for the A-V sequential delay.

3. The bifocal demand pacemaker can stimulate both atria and ventricles in sequence, it can stimulate the atria alone, or it can remain totally dormant. Thus the pacemaker functions automatically according to the patient's needs.

4. In general, the bifocal demand pacemaker is indicated in the following situations:

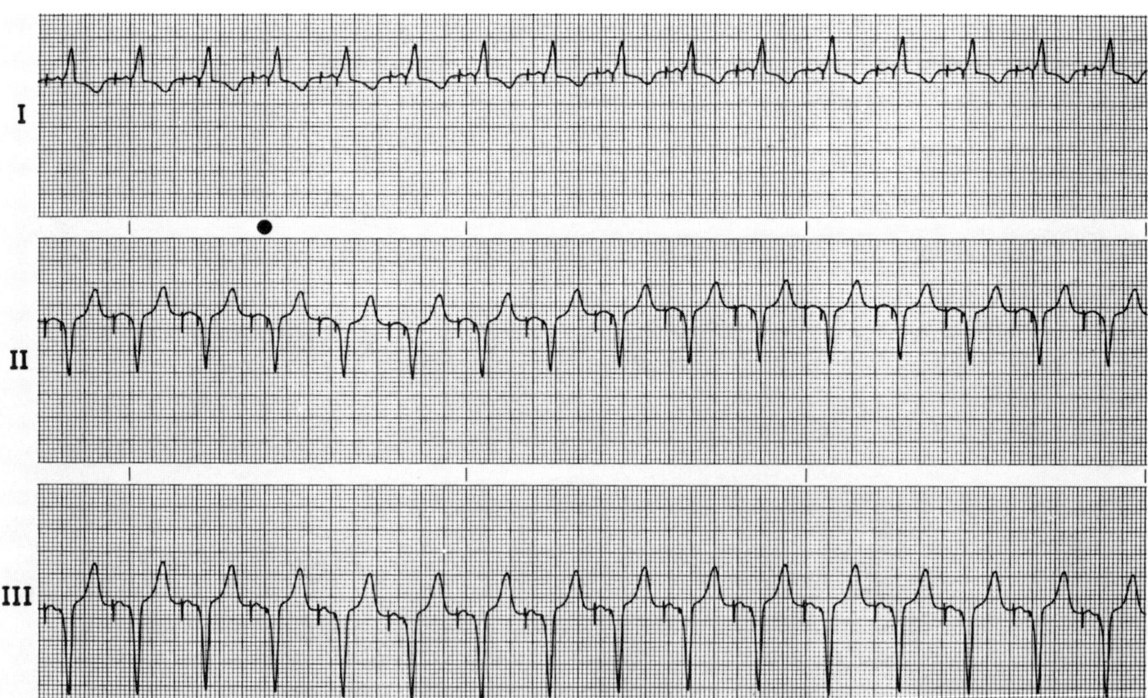

FIGURE 1-5. Bifocal demand pacemaker rhythm with a rate of 97 beats/min. Note that there are two sets of artificial pacemaker spikes. One pacemaker spike precedes the P wave, and another precedes the QRS complex.

1. SSS
2. Significant atrial bradyarrhythmias associated with intermittent high degree or complete A-V block (symptomatic)
3. High degree or complete A-V block (symptomatic), in that the atrial contribution to the ventricular output is essential

5. The bifocal demand pacemaker does not compete with spontaneous ventricular contractions.

Multiprogrammable Pacemakers

1. The purpose of multiprogrammability of artificial pacing is to provide optimal cardiac function to an individual with a specific clinical circumstance by modifying and controlling various pacemaker parameters (functions) noninvasively after pacemaker implantation.

2. The idea of the programmability of artificial pacing was introduced as early as 1960, but modern programmable pacemakers were first seen in early 1973. Initially, only two pacemaker functions (pacing rate and energy output) were programmed.

3. Newer multiprogrammable pacemakers have the capability of modifying many parameters, including:

Pacing rate
Energy output (pulse amplitude or duration)
Sensitivity (sensing threshold)
Refractory period
Hysteresis
Pacing mode
A-V delay

4. Nine of 14 pacemaker manufacturers which produce artificial pacemakers in the United States provide models with multiprogrammability.

5. The pacing rate can be adjusted from 30 to 120 beats/min (up to 400 beats/min in some temporary pacing models).

6. The programmable pacemaker is very useful in patients with SSS and bradytachyarrhythmia syndrome (Figure 1-6) because it selects the optimal pacing rate for the patient's exact need.

7. In elderly individuals and patients with angina pectoris, a relatively slow pacing rate is desirable. Depending on the patient's cardiac status, the pacing rate may have to be increased or reduced.

8. Overdrive pacing is indicated for refractory tachyarrhythmias. In this case, the best effective pacing rate may be selected noninvasively for the patient's need.

9. The energy source for the multiprogrammable pacemaker is lithium, which usually lasts 10 to 12 years.

10. Disadvantageous aspects of the programmable pacemaker include the following:

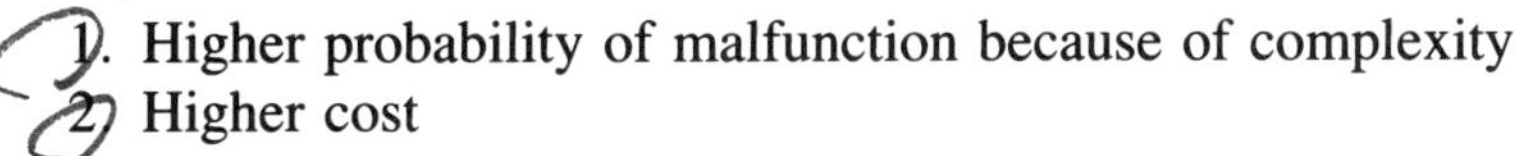

1. Higher probability of malfunction because of complexity
2. Higher cost

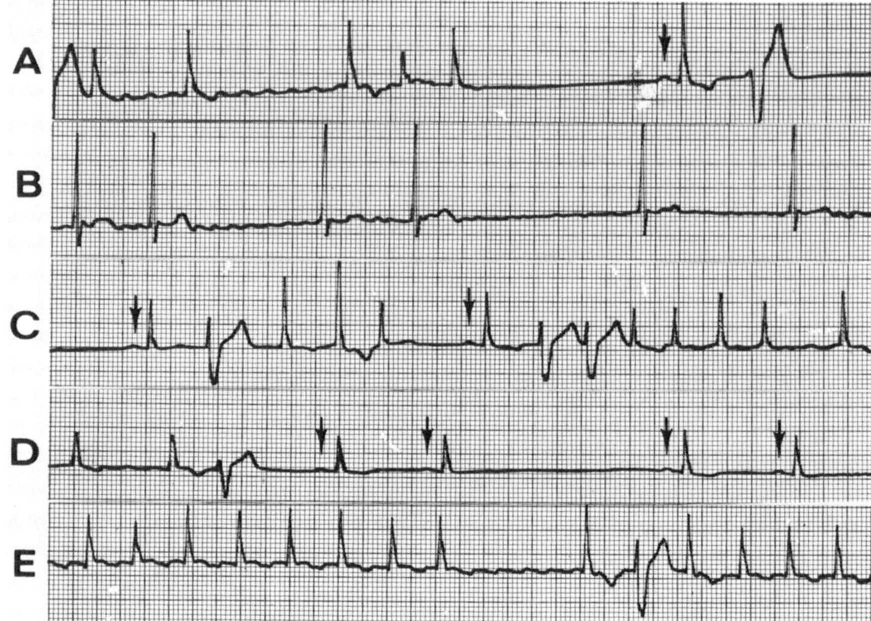

FIGURE 1-6. These Holter monitor ECG rhythm strips A to E are not continuous. The rhythm is a very unstable sinus bradycardia (*arrows*) with intermittent atrial flutter and frequent VPCs as well as aberrant ventricular conduction. These findings represent bradytachyarrhythmia syndrome as a manifestation of advanced SSS.

3. Greater educational burdens for physicians, technicians, and all involved personnel because of complex design
4. Increased reluctance of all cardiac patients with programmable pacemakers to take a trip overseas or to small towns where sophisticated medical facilities and highly trained cardiologists or cardiac surgeons are not readily available

Miscellaneous Remarks

The pacing site may be in the atria or coronary sinus region in order to utilize the atrial contribution and normal activation of the entire heart. In *coronary sinus pacemaker rhythm*, the retrograde P wave is initiated by the pacing spike and followed by the optimal P-R interval and normal QRS complex (Figure 1-7).

Nuclear-powered artificial pacemakers were introduced into clinical medicine more than a decade ago, particularly in many European countries, but they are infrequently used today because they have no clear advantage over pacemakers with a lithium energy source. In addition, the usual problems associated with the nuclear-powered pacemaker prevent its usage in clinical medicine.

COMPLICATIONS OF ARTIFICIAL PACING

During the insertion or implantation of an artificial pacemaker, the danger of inducing VF is always possible; therefore a cardioverter must be immediately available. In addition, various commonly used antiarrhythmic agents also should be at hand. Common complications are as follows.

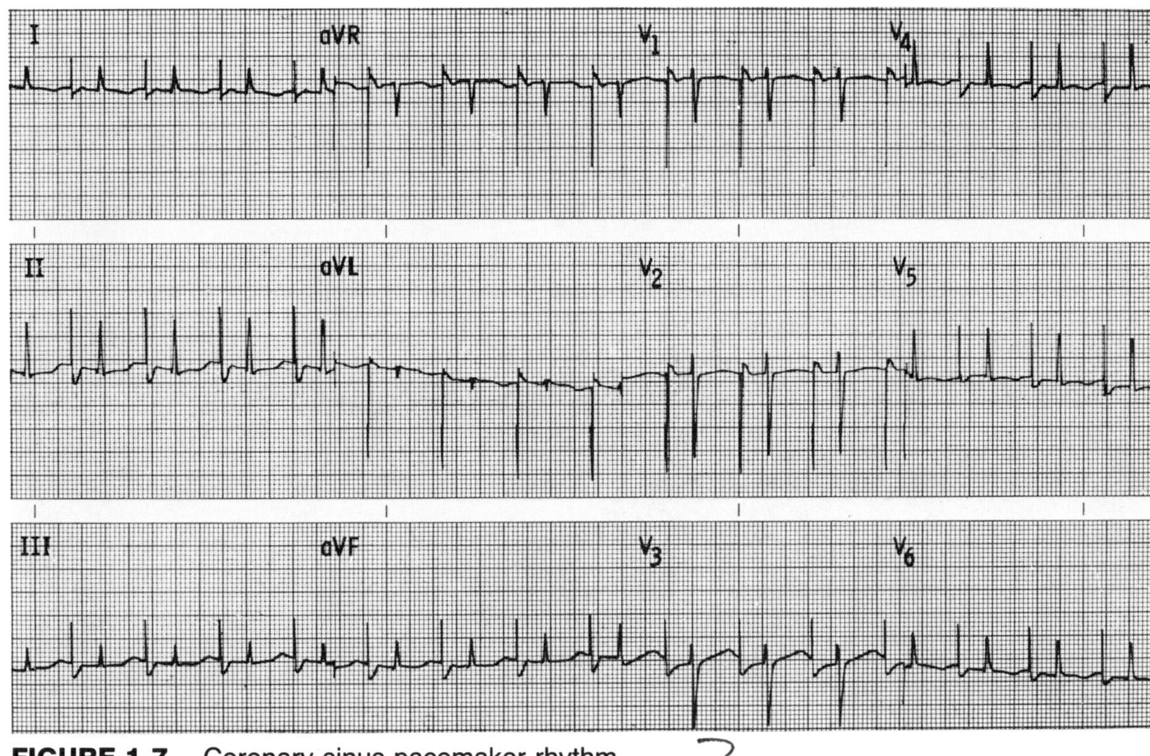

FIGURE 1-7. Coronary sinus pacemaker rhythm.

Malfunctioning Artificial Pacemakers

A malfunctioning unit (see Chapter 11) may manifest its problems in the following ways.

Acceleration of Pacing Rate (Runaway Pacemaker)

1. Runaway pacemaker is common when a fixed-rate pacemaker is used.

2. When the runaway pacemaker runs extremely fast, the preexisting bradyarrhythmia reappears.

3. VF may occur in advanced cases of runaway pacemaker, although it can also occur even with a normally functioning pacemaker.

4. Runaway pacemaker is a medical emergency. The malfunctioning unit should be promptly disconnected from the heart, which can be accomplished by cutting the electrode wires near their attachment to the pacer. Connecting a temporary pacemaker to the bare electrode ends usually results in prompt recovery.

5. Antitachyarrhythmic agents are ineffective for runaway pacemaker.

Slowing of Pacing Rate

1. Slowing of the pacing rate is a common form of malfunction when a demand unit is used.

2. It may be associated with irregular pacing.

Irregular Pacing

1. Irregular pacing is usually observed in an advanced or late state of malfunction.

2. It may be associated with slowing or acceleration of the pacing rate.

Failure of Cardiac Capture

1. Failure of cardiac capture is a very common problem.

2. It may be associated with runaway pacemaker or slowing of the pacing rate.

3. Failure of capture may occur in a normally functioning pacemaker for various reasons (e.g., quinidine or procainamide toxicity, hyperkalemia, advanced underlying heart disease).

Failure of Sensing

1. Failure of sensing may occur alone, but it often coexists with failure of cardiac capture.

2. It may be associated with other manifestations of malfunction.

3. Failure of sensing may also occur in normally functioning pacemakers for various reasons (e.g., low amplitude of QRS complex of the natural beats).

Perforation of the Ventricles

1. Perforation of the ventricles can occur when a transverse catheter electrode is used.

2. It may be suspected when the following findings occur unexpectedly:

- Right bundle branch block (RBBB)
- Recurrent diaphragmatic contraction
- Pericarditis or pericardial effusions
- Pansystolic murmur (due to rupture of the ventricular septum)

Other Findings

1. Electrode fracture
2. Infection
3. Thrombosis or embolism
4. Knotting of the wire
5. Various cardiac arrhythmias which may be due to malfunction of the unit or which may simply coexist with the normally functioning pacemaker rhythm

POSSIBLE INTERFERENCE WITH ARTIFICIAL PACEMAKER FUNCTION

The following may interfere with artificial pacemaker function:

1. Electric shavers
2. Automobile motors
3. Motorcycles

4. Malfunctioning television sets
5. Ungrounded electrical appliance (direct contact)
6. Equipment that produces strong, rapidly fluctuating magnetic fields (indirect interference by proximity)
7. Muscle stimulator for home use
8. Electric motors fitted with brushes and commutators
9. Motor-operated hospital beds
10. Electrosurgical and physical therapy equipment
11. Direct current shock

FACTORS MODIFYING PACEMAKER FUNCTION

There are various factors that may modify artificial pacemaker function:

1. Sympathomimetic amines may increase myocardial irritability.
2. Hyperkalemia may cause failure of cardiac capture.
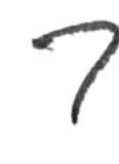
3. Fibrosis around the pacemaker electrode may cause failure of cardiac capture.
4. Advancement of underlying heart disease may cause failure of cardiac capture.
5. Quinidine or procainamide toxicity may cause failure of cardiac capture.

AFTERCARE OF PATIENTS WITH ARTIFICIAL PACEMAKERS

Chapter 12 discusses more fully the aftercare of patients with artificial pacemakers.

Patient Responsibilities

1. Every patient with a permanent pacemaker should check the pulse once or twice daily to be certain the pacemaker's preset rate remains constant.

2. In case of an altered pulse rate (either decreased or increased), the physician should be notified immediately because this may be an indication of pacemaker malfunction.

3. When any new symptoms or signs (e.g., chest pain, syncopal episodes, dizziness, or wound infection) occur, the physician should be notified immediately.

Physician Responsibilities

1. After pacemaker implantation and before the patient is discharged, the patient should be fully instructed regarding the *usual daily care* of the pacemaker, including common signs of a malfunction.

2. The patient should be given an *identification card* indicating: his or her name, the date of pacemaker implantation, the name of the surgeon who performed the implantation and/or the physician who will follow the patient after discharge, the name of the institution where the pace-

maker was implanted, the type and model number of the pacemaker and the manufacturer's name, and a medical summary, including medications being taken (optional).

3. *Pacemaker follow-up care*

1. First visit (1 month after discharge)
   a. Check surgical wound.
   b. Detect gross evidence of malfunction.
   c. Ask usual pulse rate and any complaint, e.g., chest pain or syncopal episode.
2. Routine visit (every 3 to 6 months): Perform such procedures as ECG analysis.
3. Elective hospitalization: for a battery change.
4. Emergency hospitalization: for replacing a malfunctioning unit.

4. *Pacemaker follow-up procedure for each visit*

1. Complete check-up of patient's cardiac status and status of pacemaker implantation site and the pacemaker function.
2. Long rhythm strips (leads II and V_2) to check the pacing rate and to compare with preset rate.
3. A 12-lead ECG (at least once or twice a year) to detect any unexpected or new ECG abnormality.
4. When the patient's own sinus rhythm returns after implantation of a demand pacemaker, certain maneuvers [e.g., reducing the patient's own heart rate by carotid sinus stimulation or by edrophonium chloride (Tensilon) injection, or by accelerating the artificial pacemaker rate by using a magnet] should enable one to check the function of the pacemaker.
5. Ask about any unusual or new complaint, e.g., chest pain or fainting episodes.
6. Arrange elective or emergency surgery as needed.

5. *ECG analysis of pacemaker function*

1. Long rhythm strip (lead II) and preferably a six-lead ECG at each visit.
2. A 12-lead ECG every 12 months (routine checkup) when malfunction is suspected and when the patient has unusual or new symptoms.
3. Measure pacing rate to compare with preset rate.
4. Measure pacemaker artifact amplitude to compare with preset amplitude (often special equipment is needed).
5. Detect cardiac arrhythmias.

6. *Radiographic analysis of pacemaker function*

1. Chest radiographs (and sometimes films of the abdomen) are taken before discharge, 6 to 9 months after discharge, and yearly thereafter. Films should also be taken immediately when malfunction is suspected.
2. Check the position of the pacemaker and lead system. Malposition, twisting, angulation, and rotation of the electrode or pulse generator should be checked.

7. *Pacemaker clinic*

1. When a pacemaker clinic with a specially designed pacemaker follow-up device is available, various pacemaker functions can be tested. This can be done on each patient's visit to the clinic.
2. Follow-up care can be provided through a long-distance telephone (a specially designed transtelephonic monitoring system).
3. Various pacemaker functions (e.g., pacing rate and energy output) can be adjusted as needed when the pacemaker has multiprogrammable capability.

A-V Conduction Disturbances

2

Conduction disturbances may occur anywhere in the heart and are ordinarily expressed as a "block." In general, impairment of conduction is divided into four major categories according to the location of the block: (1) sinoatrial (S-A) block (conduction disturbance at the sinoatrial junctional tissue); (2) intraatrial block (conduction disturbance within the atria); (3) atrioventricular (A-V) block (conduction disturbance at the A-V junctional tissue); and (4) intraventricular block (conduction disturbance within the ventricles). Recent electrophysiological studies have demonstrated that a block may also occur within the His bundle. Among these conduction disturbances, A-V block is the most common and may be associated with a block anywhere else in the heart. Although a common definition of A-V block is a conduction disturbance occurring at the A-V junction, the term "heart block" has been used loosely to designate A-V block.

Delayed conduction from the atria to the ventricles was recognized as early as 1899 by Wenckebach and subsequently in 1906 by Hay. Wenckebach specifically observed a gradual lengthening of the a-c intervals of the jugular pulse followed by a dropped pulse. This type of A-V block was later termed "Wenckebach A-V block" after the man who first described it. The same author also observed another type of second degree A-V block without a gradual lengthening of the a-c interval. However, the dropped pulse was initially considered to be due to decreased ventricular excitability rather than to impaired conduction at the A-V junction. Subsequently, in 1924, after the introduction of the electrocardiogram (ECG), a progressive lengthening of the P-R interval followed by a blocked P wave was described by Mobitz. Mobitz also described another type of second degree A-V block which produced a blocked P wave without a gradual lengthening of the P-R intervals. The former type of second degree A-V block is commonly called Mobitz type I A-V block or Wenckebach A-V block, whereas the latter type is termed

Mobitz type II A-V block. Thus two types of second degree A-V block are named after their describers.

A-V block is characterized by an abnormally prolonged A-V conduction time (P-R interval) or failure of conduction of one or more atrial impulses (either sinus or ectopic) because of a prolonged refractory period in the A-V node, bundle of His, and/or bilateral bundle branch system. Thus true A-V block must be distinguished from functional A-V block, which occurs as a physiological mechanism. For example, when a sinus P wave which falls outside the Q-T interval of the preceding ventricular beat fails to conduct to the ventricles or conducts slowly (P-R interval of 0.21 sec or longer), a true A-V block is said to be present. On the other hand, atrial flutter with 2:1 A-V conduction commonly occurs because of a functional rather than a true A-V block. This occurs because the A-V junctional tissue is unable to respond to the rapid atrial rate as a result of its longer refractory period. For a similar reason, the P wave of the atrial premature contraction (APC) often fails to conduct to the ventricles when the P wave appears soon after the QRS complex of the preceding beat. The P-R interval of an atrial premature contraction becomes prolonged when the P wave falls in the second half of the Q-T interval of the preceding beat. These alterations of the A-V conduction in an APC are functional (physiological) and therefore are *not* a manifestation of a true A-V block.

It has been shown that the normal absolute refractory period of the A-V junctional tissue corresponds approximately to the initial half of the Q-T interval, whereas the relative refractory period corresponds to the second half of the Q-T interval. In general, the duration of the refractory period of the A-V junction is directly related to the length of the preceding cardiac cycle. Thus it can be said that the longer the preceding cycle length, the longer is the duration of the refractory period of the beat after that cycle, whereas the shorter the preceding cycle the shorter is the duration of the refractory period. This finding is termed Ashman's phenomenon.

CLASSIFICATION

A-V block is divided into two major categories: incomplete (partial) and complete. Incomplete A-V block includes first, second, and high degree (advanced) A-V blocks, but the term is most often loosely used to designate second degree A-V block. A-V block may occur transiently, intermittently, or permanently, and one type may change to another from time to time in the same individual. In general, the following classification of A-V block is used according to the degree of the A-V conduction disturbance (Table 2-1).

First Degree A-V Block

First degree A-V block is characterized by a prolonged P-R interval (0.21 sec or more in adults and 0.18 sec or more in children) in which every atrial impulse reaches the ventricles with constant P-R intervals.

TABLE 2-1. A-V Block: Classification

First degree A-V block
Second degree A-V block
Wenckebach (Mobitz type I) A-V block
Mobitz type II A-V block
2:1 A-V block
High degree (advanced) A-V block
Complete (third degree) A-V block

Second Degree A-V Block

Second degree A-V block is diagnosed when some of the atrial impulses fail to reach the ventricles so that QRS complexes are unexpectedly absent. Atrioventricular ratios are used to compare the number of impulses conducted to the atria with those conducted to the ventricles. For instance, 4:3 A-V block indicates that for every four atrial impulses three are conducted to the ventricles. There are two types of second degree A-V block. The common type is called Wenckebach (Mobitz type I) second degree A-V block, in which the P-R interval of each successively conducted beat lengthens progressively until a P wave is not followed by a QRS complex (blocked P wave). The uncommon type is characterized by the occurrence of a blocked P wave and otherwise constant P-R intervals in all conducted beats (Mobitz type II A-V block). A-V ratios may be 3:2, 4:3, 5:4, 6:5, etc. in either Mobitz type I or II A-V block. The A-V ratio may be fixed or may vary throughout the tracing. A 2:1 A-V block is diagnosed when every other atrial impulse is blocked, and it may be a variant of either Mobitz type I or II A-V block.

Advanced (High Degree) A-V Block

Advanced A-V block is diagnosed when a blocked P wave occurs in more than a 2:1 A-V ratio. Thus 3:1, 4:1, 5:1, 6:1, etc. A-V blocks belong to this category. A-V ratios of the even numbers, e.g., 4:1 or 6:1 A-V block, are much more common than those of the odd numbers, e.g., 3:1 or 5:1 A-V block. In advanced A-V block, A-V junctional escape beats (less commonly ventricular escape beats) frequently appear as a physiological mechanism, leading to incomplete A-V dissociation.

Complete (Third Degree) A-V Block

Complete A-V block indicates that none of the atrial impulses are conducted to the ventricles. Consequently, in almost every case the A-V junctional escape rhythm or, less commonly, the ventricular escape (idioventricular) rhythm seems to control the ventricles. In complete A-V block, atrial and ventricular activities are independent, leading to complete A-V dissociation.

In addition, A-V conduction disturbances are further altered when there is bilateral bundle branch block (BBBB) (see Chapter 3). In fact, BBBB of different degrees may produce identical ECG findings as first, second, and third degree A-V blocks. It has been pointed out that Mobitz type II A-V block is caused by BBBB and is frequently a precursor of complete A-V block as a result of complete trifascicular block (TFB). Paroxysmal complete A-V block has been reported recently, and its occurrence was thought to be related to phase 4 BBBB. An A-V conduction disturbance is frequently bidirectional, but it may be unidirectional. For example, antegrade A-V conduction may be impaired in the presence of normal retrograde V-A conduction or vice versa. Electrophysiological studies have demonstrated recently that a pseudo-A-V block may be produced as a result of concealed His bundle premature beats.

FIRST DEGREE A-V BLOCK

First degree A-V block is the most common conduction disturbance, occurring in apparently healthy subjects as well as in those with diseased hearts. First degree A-V block is extremely common in elderly individuals without clinical evidence of heart disease. On the other hand, first degree A-V block may be observed in acute myocarditis, acute diaphragmatic myocardial infarction (MI), and mild digitalis intoxication (DI). First degree A-V block is considered to be the most common and earliest finding in acute rheumatic fever in children.

Diagnostic Criteria

1. The diagnostic feature of first degree A-V block is a prolongation of the P-R interval. Thus first degree A-V block is diagnosed when the P-R interval is 0.21 sec or longer in adults or 0.18 sec or longer in children.

2. In first degree A-V block, each atrial impulse must be conducted to the ventricles.

3. In general, the P-R intervals are constant throughout, but they may be altered in length when there is a significant change in heart rate.

4. The P-R interval after a long preceding cardiac cycle may be longer, and the P-R interval following a short preceding cardiac cycle may be shorter. This occurs because the refractory period of the A-V junctional tissue is directly influenced by the cardiac cycle of the preceding beat.

5. The P-R interval may be prolonged as much as 0.80 sec; extremely rarely, it may exceed the length of the P-P cycle. In the latter case, two P waves may precede the QRS complex, and of these two P waves the first one is conducted to the ventricles. The P wave immediately preceding the QRS complex may be either blocked or conducted to the next QRS complex. This phenomenon is termed "skipped" P wave.

Mechanism

1. In the majority of cases, first degree A-V block is considered to be caused by prolongation of the relative refractory period in the A-V

junction which extends to the end of the cycle. The prolonged refractory period is more marked in the earlier portion of the cardiac cycle.

2. Less commonly, the P-R interval may be prolonged when conduction in the common (A-V) bundle is impaired.

3. Impaired conduction in the left and right bundle branches of equal degree also produces a prolonged P-R interval.

4. When the impairment of conductivity in the right and left bundle branches is unequal in degree, a prolonged P-R interval of varying degree, associated with a QRS complex of varying configuration, may result.

5. On the other hand, a wide P wave caused either by marked left atrial enlargement or an intraatrial conduction defect also produces a prolonged P-R interval.

Clinical Significance

1. First degree A-V block may be observed in apparently healthy individuals, but it is more commonly found in diseased hearts.

2. Elderly individuals without demonstrable heart disease often have first degree A-V block which is considered to be due to chronic degenerative changes in the A-V conduction system. Therefore isolated first degree A-V block in elderly subjects (above age 60) is clinically insignificant.

3. However, first degree A-V block with acute onset is commonly caused by DI, acute diaphragmatic MI, and acute myocarditis.

4. Less commonly, first degree A-V block may be caused by hyperkalemia and uremia.

5. Chronic first degree A-V block is often followed by atrial fibrillation (AF), particularly in elderly individuals, and the finding is frequently a manifestation of the sick sinus syndrome (SSS) (see Chapter 4).

6. Treatment of first degree A-V block per se is usually not indicated, but the underlying cause (e.g., DI) must be corrected if possible.

7. Any patient with first degree A-V block of recent onset should be observed closely for possible development of a higher degree A-V block.

SECOND DEGREE A-V BLOCK

The term "incomplete A-V block" has been loosely used to designate second degree A-V block without specifying its degree or type. Thus the term incomplete A-V block often implies that it is second degree A-V block. However, the type and A-V conduction ratio should be specified in second degree A-V block because the fundamental mechanisms and their clinical significance are often different.

Second degree A-V block was initially described independently in 1899 by Wenckebach and in 1906 by Hay. Subsequently, second degree A-V block was divided into two major categories in 1924 by Mobitz.

He called the two categories Mobitz types I and II. Mobitz type I A-V block has also been called Wenckebach A-V block to distinguish it from Mobitz type II A-V block.

Second degree A-V block is diagnosed when a P wave (either sinus or ectopic) is blocked in spite of the fact that the absolute refractory period of the A-V junction is expected to be over physiologically. In other words, a P wave is not followed by QRS-T complexes because of an abnormally prolonged refractory period in the A-V junction. Mobitz type I (Wenckebach) A-V block is characterized by a progressive lengthening of the P-R intervals until a blocked P wave occurs. The occurrence of a blocked P wave, preceded by a progressive lengthening of the P-R intervals, is termed Wenckebach phenomenon or period. It should be noted that Wenckebach phenomenon may occur anywhere in the heart. On the other hand, Mobitz type II A-V block is characterized by the occurrence of a blocked P wave without the preceding Wenckebach period.

The blocked P wave may occur occasionally or frequently, periodically, and regularly or irregularly. The ratio of the A-V conduction is expressed according to the number of the P waves versus the number of the conducted QRS complexes. For example, when one of four atrial impulses is blocked, the A-V ratio is expressed as 4:3 A-V block.

Second degree A-V block occurs when the refractory periods of the A-V junctional tissue, both absolute and relative, are abnormally prolonged but do not occupy the entire cardiac cycle. In Mobitz type I (Wenckebach) A-V block, the absolute and relative refractory periods of the A-V junction are said to be prolonged to an equal or unequal degree. On the other hand, incomplete trifascicular (infranodal) block is thought to be responsible for the production of Mobitz type II A-V block (see Chapter 3).

The 2:1 A-V block is another form of second degree A-V block which may be a variant of either Mobitz type I or II A-V block.

Occasionally, second degree A-V block changes from one type to another on the same ECG tracing. Two or more consecutively appearing blocked P waves (e.g., 3:1 or 4:1 A-V block) is termed high degree or advanced A-V block. The His bundle ECG findings on A-V block are summarized in Table 2-2.

TABLE 2-2. A-V Block: His Bundle ECG Findings

A-V nodal block
- Prolonged A-H interval (normal: 50–140 msec)
- A-deflection not followed by H-deflection
- H-V interval: normal

Intra-His block
- Split H-H′ deflections > 25 msec
- A-H deflections not followed by H′-V deflections
- A-H interval: normal
- H′-V interval: often prolonged

Infra-His (infranodal) block
- Prolonged H-V interval (normal: 35–55 msec)
- A-H deflections not followed by V-deflection
- A-H interval: normal

Diagnostic Criteria

Mobitz Type I A-V Block (Wenckebach A-V Block)

Mobitz type I A-V block (Wenckebach A-V block) is a rather common form of second degree A-V block. It is diagnosed when the P-R intervals become progressively prolonged until a P wave is not followed by a QRS complex (Table 2-3).

P-R Intervals. Wenckebach A-V block is characterized by a progressive lengthening of the P-R intervals until a blocked P wave occurs. After the blocked P wave, the same cycle is repeated (Figure 2-1). The P-R interval after the pause (blocked P wave) is the shortest of all and may be within normal limits or longer than 0.20 sec. Conversely, the P-R interval immediately preceding the blocked P wave is the longest which occurs during the Wenckebach period. The maximal increment in the P-R interval occurs between the first and second conducted beats after the pause, and the increment in the length of the P-R intervals becomes less and less thereafter until the blocked P wave occurs (Figure 2-1). The fundamental mechanism responsible for alteration of the P-R intervals in Wenckebach A-V block is discussed later in the chapter (see Mechanism). Occasionally, a characteristic feature of the Wenckebach period is altered.

A-V Conduction Ratio. The A-V conduction ratio in the Wenckebach A-V block may be fixed (Figure 2-1), or it may change from time to time. Common A-V conduction ratios are either 3:2 or 4:3 A-V block, indicating that every two of three or three of four atrial impulses are conducted to the ventricles, respectively (Figure 2-1). Less commonly, the A-V conduction ratio may be 5:4, 6:5, 7:6, 8:7, etc. When the A-V conduction ratio is fixed, the ventricular rhythm shows a regular irregularity (Figure 2-1). On the other hand, the ventricular rhythm is markedly irregular when the A-V conduction ratios vary in Wenckebach A-V block. Wenckebach A-V block may transform to 2:1 A-V block from time to time.

R-R Intervals. A characteristic R-R cycle is observed during the Wenckebach period. Needless to say, the R-R interval, which includes

TABLE 2-3. Second Degree A-V Block: ECG Findings

Parameter	A-V Nodal Block	Infranodal Block
Type of block	Usually Wenckebach type (Mobitz type I) Less commonly 2:1 A-V block (variant of Wenckebach type)	Usually Mobitz type II Less commonly 2:1 A-V block (variant of Mobitz type II)
QRS contour	Almost always normal Rarely abnormal because of preexisting bundle branch block, hemiblocks, or bifascicular block	Almost always abnormal (bundle branch block, hemiblocks, or bifascicular block) Rarely normal
Nature of A-V conduction	Often normal A-V conduction returns	Common precursor of complete A-V block (complete trifascicular block)

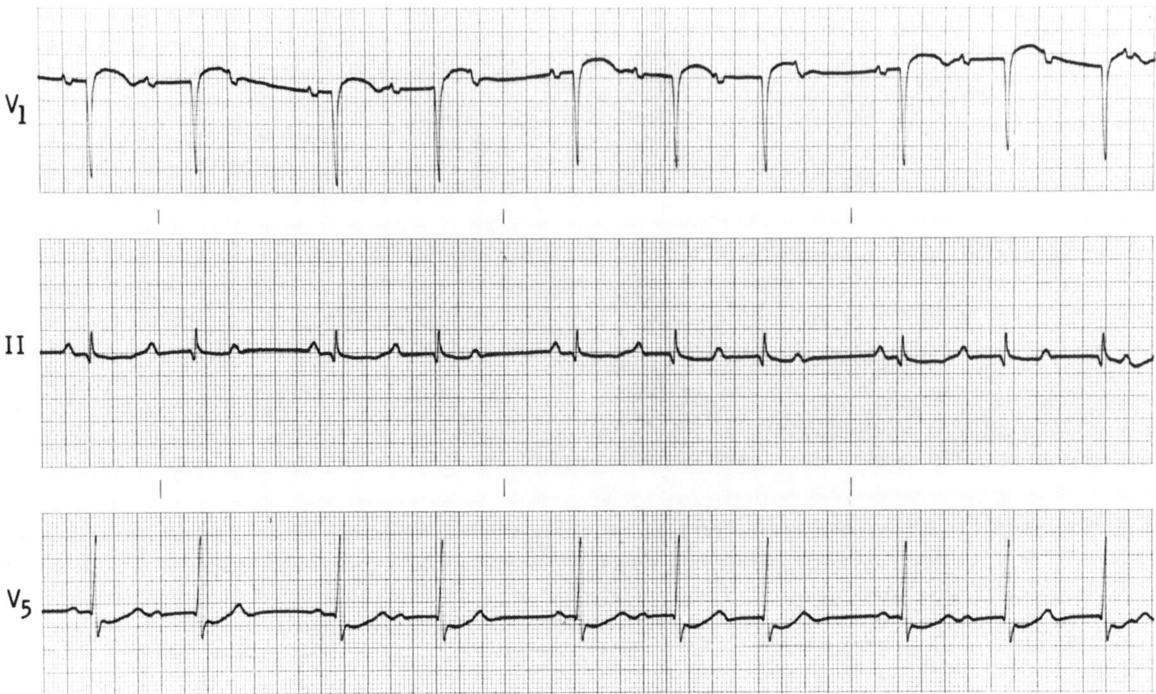

FIGURE 2-1. Sinus rhythm with Wenckebach (Mobitz type I) A-V block (3:2 and 4:3 A-V conduction ratios).

the blocked P wave, is the longest found during the Wenckebach period, but it is shorter than two cycles of the P-P interval (Figure 2-1). This occurs because the R-R interval, including the blocked P wave, is actually two P-P intervals minus the decrement in the P-R interval between the conducted sinus beats before and after the pause (Figure 2-1). The R-R interval immediately after the pause is the second longest during the Wenckebach period because of the maximal increment in the P-R interval. The R-R intervals thereafter become shorter and shorter in successively conducted beats because the degree of the increment in the P-R intervals become less and less until a blocked P wave occurs. When the A-V conduction ratio is fixed, the ventricular rhythm characteristically shows a regular irregularity (Figure 2-1). Ventricular pseudobigeminy results when the A-V conduction ratio is 3:2.

Atrial Mechanism. The atrial mechanism is commonly a sinus, but it may be atrial tachycardia or flutter. In the latter case, the Wenckebach phenomenon may be functional (physiological) due to the extremely rapid atrial rate because of the longer refractory period in the A-V junction. Rarely, A-V junctional tachycardia with Wenckebach A-V block is observed.

P-P Intervals. The P-P intervals are regular in Wenckebach A-V block but may be irregular when ordinary sinus arrhythmia is present. In addition, the P-P intervals may become periodically irregular when ventriculophasic sinus arrhythmia exists.

Configuration of the QRS Complex. In general, the QRS complex in Wenckebach A-V block is normal in configuration, but it may be bizarre and broad because of aberrant ventricular conduction or a preexisting bundle branch block.

Mobitz Type II A-V Block

Mobitz type II A-V block is a much less common form of second degree A-V block than the Wenckebach (Mobitz type I) A-V block. Mobitz type II A-V block is diagnosed when blocked P waves occur periodically without a preceding Wenckebach phenomenon (Table 2-3; Figure 2-2). When 2:1 A-V block persists, a specification of Mobitz types I and II is not always possible unless a transitional change from or to a lesser degree (3:2) A-V block or higher degree (3:1, 4:1, etc.) A-V block with occasional ventricular captured beats is observed in the same ECG tracing. Measurement of the P-R intervals of the conducted beats or of the ventricular captured beats may clarify the type of A-V block. However, in a practical sense, 2:1 A-V block associated with bundle branch blocks, hemiblocks, or bifascicular block (BFB) is a variant of Mobitz type II A-V block (Figure 2-3).

P-R Intervals. The P-R intervals of all the conducted beats in Mobitz type II A-V block are usually constant (Figure 2-2). The P-R intervals in conducted beats in 2:1 A-V block are usually constant, but they may be normal or prolonged.

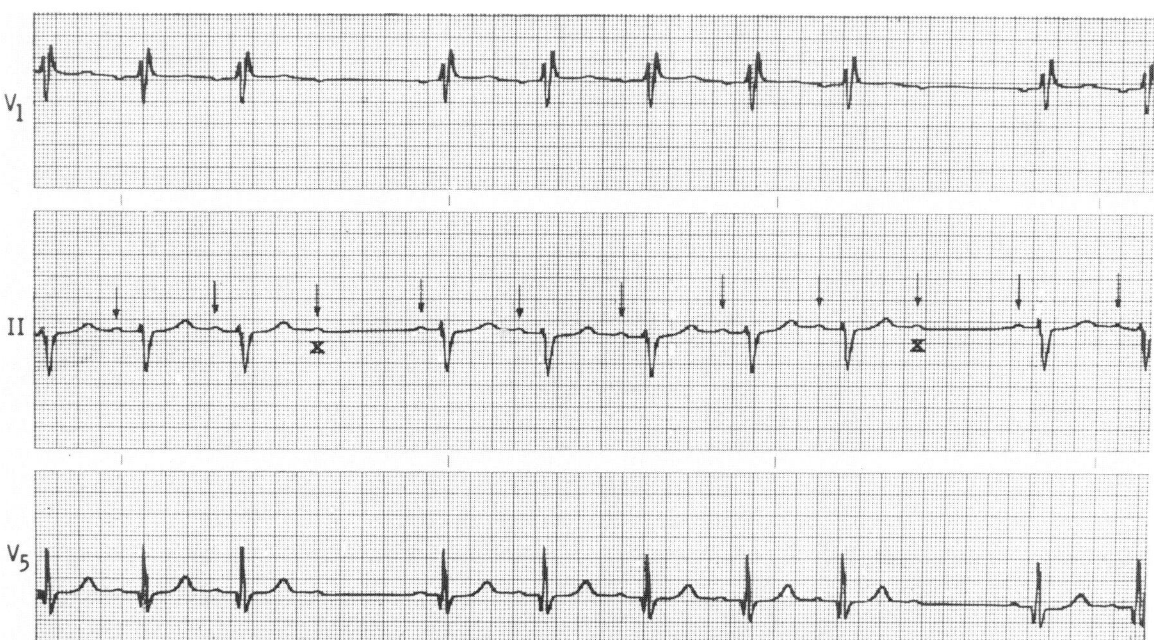

FIGURE 2-2. Sinus rhythm (*arrows*) with intermittent Mobitz type II A-V block. Note the occasional blocked sinus P waves (*X*). The diagnosis of BFB (a combination of RBBB and left anterior hemiblock) is obvious. Therefore these ECG findings represent incomplete TFB.

A-V Conduction Ratio. The A-V conduction ratio, like that in Wenckebach A-V block, may be fixed or may vary. The A-V ratio is commonly 3:2 or 4:3, and less commonly 5:4, 6:5, 7:6, 8:7, etc. A-V conduction may be observed. Mobitz type II A-V block (i.e., 3:2 or 4:3 A-V block) may change to or from 2:1 A-V block.

R-R Intervals. The R-R intervals, including the blocked P wave, are usually multiples of the P-P interval (the basic sinus cycle).

P-P Intervals. The P-P intervals in Mobitz type II A-V block are constant unless sinus arrhythmia exists. On the other hand, short and long P-P intervals may occur alternatively in 2:1 A-V block because of ventriculophasic sinus arrhythmia. In this case, the P-P interval including the QRS complex is shorter than that without the QRS complex. On rare occasions the reverse phenomenon may occur.

Atrial Mechanism. The atrial mechanism is usually sinus, and the ectopic atrial mechanism is rare.

Configuration of the QRS Complex. Mobitz type II A-V block is nearly always associated with RBBB or LBBB, hemiblocks, or BFB (Figures 2-2 and 2-3). A normal QRS complex with the Mobitz type II A-V block is rather unusual.

2:1 A-V Block

The term 2:1 A-V block is used when every other P wave is conducted to the ventricles. Although 2:1 A-V block is a variant of either Mobitz type I or II A-V block (Table 2-3), it cannot be positively diagnosed unless the transitional change from or to Mobitz type I or II A-V block is observed in the same ECG tracing. However, it can be said that 2:1 A-V block is a variant of Wenckebach (Mobitz type I) A-V block when the QRS complex exhibits a normal (narrow) contour (Figure 2-3). Conversely, 2:1 A-V block is nearly always a variant of Mobitz type II A-V block when the QRS complex reveals bundle branch block, hemiblock (left anterior or posterior), or BFB (Figure 2-3).

Mechanism

Electrophysiological studies utilizing His bundle ECG analysis regarding the mechanism of A-V block are summarized in Table 2-2.

Mobitz Type I A-V Block (Wenckebach A-V Block)

Mobitz type I A-V block is thought to be caused by prolongation of the absolute and relative refractory periods in the A-V junction to an equal or unequal degree. The characteristic feature of the Wenckebach phenomenon (progressive lengthening of P-R intervals until a blocked P wave occurs) is explained as follows (Figure 2-4).

1. The maximal increment of the P-R interval occurs in the second conducted beat after the pause. This is observed because the refractory period of the A-V junction is directly related to the length of the preceding R-R interval; that is, the longest R-R interval (pause) induces a marked increase in the length of the refractory period in the A-V junction

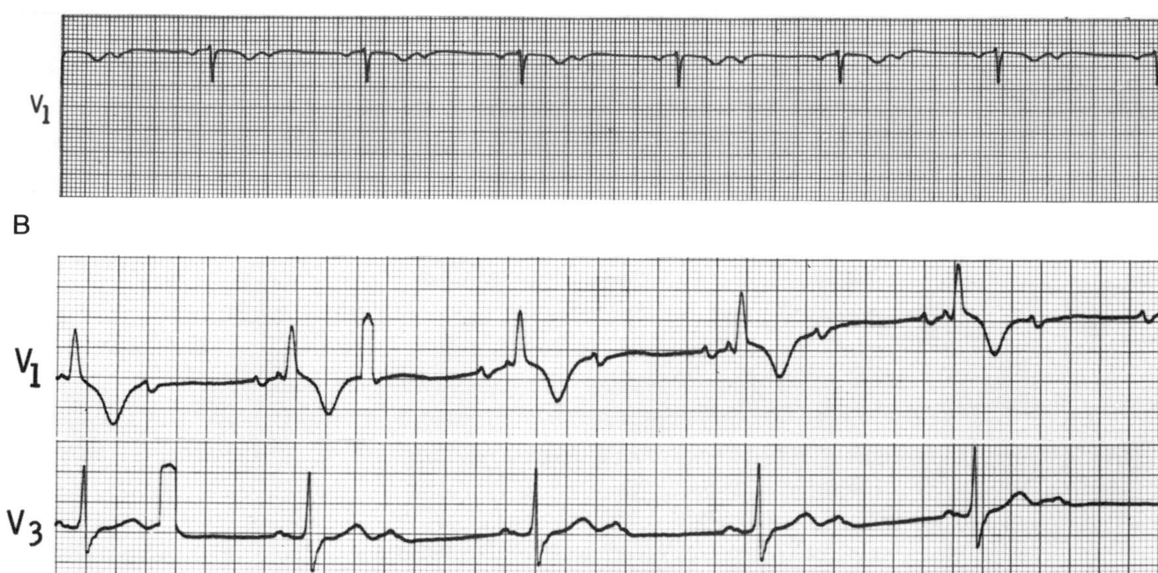

FIGURE 2-3. **A:** Sinus rhythm with 2:1 A-V block (most likely A-V nodal block). **B:** Sinus rhythm with 2:1 A-V block and RBBB (most likely infranodal block).

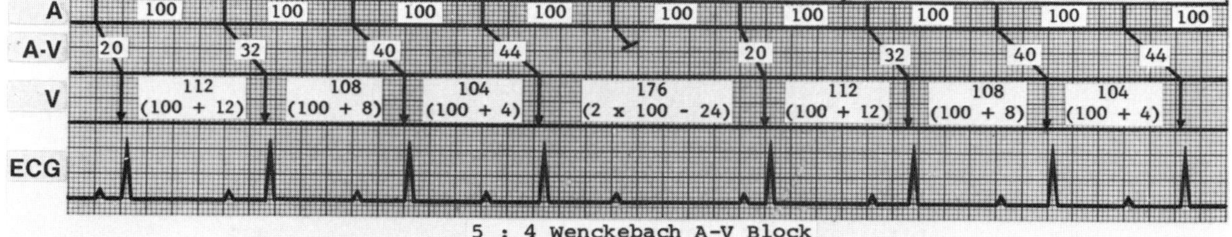

FIGURE 2-4. Mobitz type I (Wenckebach) A-V block. The numbers represent hundredths of a second. The numbers in the upper row represent the atrial cycle (P-P interval) with a rate of 60/min. The numbers within the oblique lines at the A-V level indicate the A-V conduction time (P-R interval). Progressive lengthening of the P-R intervals is apparent until a blocked atrial impulse (dropped P wave) occurs. After this blocked atrial impulse, the P-R interval shortens to its original value (0.20 sec), and the sequence is repeated. The numbers in the lower row represent the duration of successive ventricular cycles. The progressive shortening of the ventricular cycle length (R-R interval) is due to the progressive increment of A-V conduction before the blocked atrial impulse and the decrement immediately after the blocked P wave. The numbers in parentheses in the lower row indicate the degree of increment or decrement in the ventricular cycle length.

leading to a maximal increment of the P-R interval in the second conducted beat.

2. After the maximal increment of the P-R interval in the second conducted beat, the P-R intervals in the subsequent beats progressively lengthen until a blocked P wave occurs but the degree of the increment in the P-R intervals becomes less and less.

3. Consequently, the R-R intervals after the pause progressively shorten until a blocked P wave occurs. The progressive shortening of the R-R intervals is caused by two opposing effects on the refractoriness in the A-V junction. They are a shortening effect because of the shorter cycle lengths per se and a lengthening effect consequent to the increasing fatigue (refractoriness) of the A-V junctional tissue.

4. During the Wenckebach period, the R-R interval of each consecutively conducted beat is equal in length to the P-P interval plus the increment of the P-R interval between the two successively conducted beats.

5. Conversely, the R-R interval, which includes the blocked P wave (pause), is equal in length to two P-P intervals minus the decrement in the P-R interval between the conducted sinus beats before and after the pause.

6. As a result, the longest R-R interval (pause), which contains the blocked P wave, is usually shorter than two short R-R intervals or two P-P intervals.

7. For a similar reason, the R-R interval of the first beat after the pause is longer than the R-R interval of the last beat before the pause.

8. When the P-P cycles vary because of sinus arrhythmia, the above-mentioned characteristic features of Wenckebach period may be somewhat altered.

9. In addition, ventriculophasic sinus arrhythmia also may produce an alteration of the Wenckebach period.

10. Occasionally, an unexpectedly long or short P-R interval or an unexpectedly conducted or blocked P wave may occur in Wenckebach A-V block because of concealed A-V conduction and/or supernormal A-V conduction. In these circumstances, the characteristic Wenckebach period is again altered.

11. Premature contractions, particularly those which are ventricular in origin, often alter the Wenckebach period, but in most instances concealed A-V conduction is responsible.

Mobitz Type II A-V Block

Mobitz type II A-V block is characterized by the occasional occurrence of a blocked P wave without the preceding Wenckebach period (Figure 2-2).

1. It has been recently shown that an infra-A-V nodal lesion is responsible for the production of Mobitz type II A-V block.

2. In addition, various investigators strongly suggest that incomplete BBBB is often the cause of Mobitz type II A-V block.

3. In fact, Mobitz type II A-V block is frequently associated with

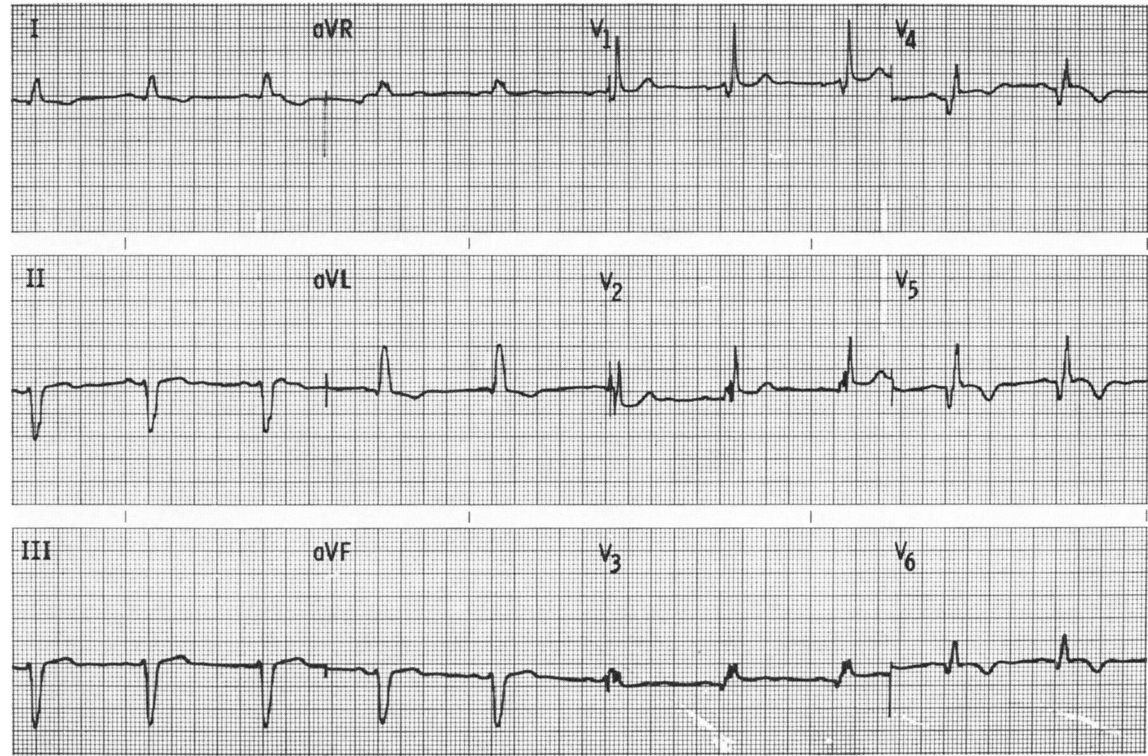

FIGURE 2-5. BFB consisting of RBBB and left anterior hemiblock due to a recent extensive anterior MI. The rhythm is sinus.

bundle branch block, particularly RBBB with left anterior hemiblock (Figure 2-5).

4. Furthermore, it has also been documented that Adams-Stokes syndrome is prone to develop in patients with Mobitz type II A-V block, and therefore it is considered to be a precursor of complete A-V block resulting from complete TFB.

5. It is not uncommon to observe that Mobitz type II A-V block transforms to high degree or complete A-V block (incomplete or complete TFB).

2:1 A-V Block

As described previously, Mobitz type I or II A-V block may cause 2:1 A-V block.

1. The mechanism responsible for the production of 2:1 A-V block as a result of Wenckebach (Mobitz type I) A-V block, needless to say, is a block in the A-V node itself (A-V nodal or intranodal block) (Figure 2-3).

2. On the other hand, 2:1 A-V block as a variant of Mobitz type II A-V block is caused by infranodal block (Table 2-3).

3. In either circumstance, every other P wave is conducted to the ventricles, leading to a slow ventricular rate (Figure 2-3).

Clinical Significance

The clinical significance of Mobitz types I and II is quite different.

1. In general, Mobitz type I A-V block (Wenckebach A-V block) produces no or very few symptoms.

2. Mobitz type II A-V block, on the other hand, is often associated with a high incidence of congestive heart failure (CHF) and/or Adams-Stokes syndrome.

3. Some sensitive patients experience palpitations or skipped heart beats which may resemble or be identical with the feeling induced by premature contractions.

4. When blocked P waves occur frequently and the ventricular rate becomes slow, particularly in Mobitz type II A-V block, patients may experience dizziness, fainting, or even complete unconsciousness.

5. Permanent artificial pacing is mandatory in all patients with Mobitz type II A-V block because of the nature of the block—infranodal block (see Chapters 3 and 8).

6. As emphasized previously, Adams-Stokes syndrome is prone to occur in patients with Mobitz type II A-V block because it is considered to be a precursor of complete A-V block resulting from complete trifascicular block (Table 2-3).

7. Mobitz type I (Wenckebach) A-V block is often transient in nature and may be induced by mild DI, acute infection (i.e., acute rheumatic fever, diphtheria, scarlet fever, and many other forms of bacterial, viral, and fungal infection), uremia, or electrolyte imbalance.

8. Acute diaphragmatic MI is often associated with Mobitz type I A-V block because of a transient ischemic change in the A-V junction. Because the commonest cause of acute diaphragmatic MI is occlusion of the right coronary artery, which also supplies the A-V junction, the infarction is often associated with Mobitz type I A-V block.

9. On the other hand, acute anteroseptal MI is commonly associated with Mobitz type II A-V block or even complete A-V block (complete trifascicular block) because of irreversible changes (necrosis) in the bifurcation, the bundle branches, or both (see Chapter 3).

10. Cardiac surgery of various types may induce a transient or permanent A-V block of varying degree.

11. Wenckebach (Mobitz type I) A-V block is not uncommon during physical exercise, especially when the atrial rate exceeds 150 beats/min.

12. In addition, Wenckebach A-V block is encountered in apparently healthy individuals on rare occasions.

13. Mobitz type I A-V block (Wenckebach A-V block) per se usually does not require treatment unless the patient is symptomatic.

14. Removal or treatment of the direct cause of the A-V block (i.e., DI, infections) is extremely important in preventing the development of a higher degree A-V block.

15. When there is CHF, it should be treated accordingly.

16. The prognosis in Mobitz type I A-V block is generally good, whereas Mobitz type II A-V block has a serious outcome.

17. The nature and severity of the underlying heart disease directly influence the prognosis.

HIGH DEGREE (ADVANCED) A-V BLOCK

High degree (advanced) A-V block is diagnosed when the A-V conduction ratio is 3:1 or more. Thus high degree A-V block is between second degree A-V block and complete A-V block; in other words, high degree A-V block is the most advanced form of incomplete A-V block. It is not uncommon to observe that complete A-V block is initiated by high degree A-V block. Common A-V conduction ratios are even-numbered (e.g., 4:1, 6:1, 8:1); odd-numbered A-V conduction ratios (e.g., 3:1, 5:1, 7:1) are relatively uncommon. Because of a slow ventricular rhythm in high degree A-V block, A-V junctional escape beats or, less commonly, ventricular escape (idioventricular) beats seem to control the ventricles as a physiological mechanism. It is the rule rather than the exception to observe one or more A-V junctional escape beats, particularly when A-V conduction ratios are 4:1 or higher. When A-V conduction ratios further increase in high degree A-V block, the numbers of the A-V junctional escape beats exceed those of the conducted beats. In this circumstance, conducted beats (ventricular captured beats) may occur very rarely; otherwise, the ECG tracing shows complete A-V block. Some investigators designate this extremely advanced A-V block as ''almost complete A-V block.''

In high degree A-V block, incomplete A-V dissociation often results because the A-V junctional escape beats (QRS complexes) and the sinus P waves are independent except for the conducted beats (ventricular captured beats). The atrial mechanism in high degree A-V block may be an ectopic rhythm, e.g., atrial fibrillation or flutter, or tachycardia.

Diagnostic Criteria

By definition, high degree (advanced) A-V block indicates that the A-V conduction ratio is 3:1 or more.

A-V Conduction Ratio

1. Common A-V conduction ratios in high degree A-V block are even numbers, e.g., 4:1, 6:1, 8:1, 10:1.

2. Less commonly, the A-V conduction ratios are odd numbers, e.g., 3:1, 5:1, 7:1.

3. When conducted beats appear only occasionally, an exact A-V conduction ratio is difficult or impossible to determine, especially when dealing with a limited length of the ECG tracing.

4. It is not uncommon to observe only one or two conducted beats (ventricular captured beats) in an entire ECG tracing. Needless to say, in this case A-V junctional escape rhythm is present to control the ventricles and is independent of the P waves, resulting in incomplete A-V dissociation. Thus the A-V block in this situation is nearly complete and has been termed ''almost complete A-V block'' by some investigators.

5. High degree or complete A-V block is one of the three major underlying rhythm disorders responsible for the production of A-V dissociation.

P-R Intervals

As seen in second degree A-V block, the P-R intervals of the conducted beats in high degree A-V block may be normal, but they may also be markedly prolonged. In general, the P-R intervals of the conducted beats are constant.

Atrial Mechanism

The atria may be controlled by the sinus node, but it is not uncommon for the atrial mechanism to be an ectopic rhythm, e.g., atrial fibrillation or flutter, or tachycardia.

A-V Dissociation

One or more A-V junctional escape beats commonly occur to control the ventricles in high degree A-V block whenever the ventricular rhythm becomes slower than that of an A-V junctional escape rhythm. This results in incomplete A-V dissociation. It is rather unusual not to observe A-V junctional escape beats in spite of an extremely slow ventricular rhythm. In this circumstance, concealed A-V conduction is considered to be responsible: the A-V junctional escape beat fails to appear because the A-V junctional pacemaker is passively discharged by the atrial impulse, which penetrates deeply into the A-V junction. Ventricular escape (idioventricular) beats rarely appear in high degree A-V block when the A-V junction is unable to function as a secondary pacemaker or the block is in the infranodal region.

P-P and R-R Intervals

1. The P-P intervals in high degree A-V block are generally regular, but they may vary when ordinary sinus arrhythmia, sinoatrial block, or ventriculophasic sinus arrhythmia is present.

2. The P-P intervals may also vary when A-V junctional premature contractions or atrial captured beats occur.

3. The R-R intervals are almost always irregular in high degree A-V block because of the frequent occurrence of A-V junctional (or ventricular) escape beats in addition to the conducted beats.

4. The R-R intervals become unexpectedly irregular when concealed A-V conduction and/or supernormal A-V conduction occurs.

5. When the A-V conduction ratio is constant, without A-V junctional escape beats, the R-R intervals are regular. The R-R intervals become irregular when the A-V conduction ratios are inconsistent.

6. When the A-V conduction ratio alternates (i.e., 2:1 alternating with 4:1 A-V conduction), ventricular pseudobigeminy results.

7. Premature contractions of various origins also produce irregular R-R intervals.

Configuration of the QRS Complex

The configuration of the QRS complex depends greatly on the origin of the QRS complex. Conducted beats usually have a normal configuration unless RBBB or LBBB is present. The QRS complex of a ventricular escape (idioventricular) beat is, needless to say, wide and bizarre. Various QRS configurations are observed when ventricular fusion beats of varying degree occur.

Mechanism

High degree (advanced) A-V block may be due to various fundamental mechanisms. As in second degree A-V block, the same mechanism responsible for the production of Mobitz type I (Wenckebach A-V block) or II A-V block may induce high degree A-V block.

1. For example, 3:1 A-V block may result from 3:2 Wenckebach A-V block. This occurs when an atrial impulse fails to conduct to the ventricles but penetrates deeply into the A-V junction (concealed A-V conduction) so that the subsequent atrial impulse finds a newly formed refractory period in the A-V junction resulting in a blocked P wave.
2. Similarly, 3:1 A-V block may be due to actual 3:2 Mobitz type II A-V block with concealed conduction in the His-Purkinje system which occurs at every third beat.
3. The above observation indicates that A-V block may be seen because of a conduction disturbance occurring at two levels in the A-V junction, including the His-Purkinje system.
4. In addition, 3:1 A-V block may be due to an uncomplicated mechanism analogous to Mobitz type II second degree A-V block.
5. Furthermore, 3:1 A-V block often results when a ventricular premature contraction (VPC) occurs in the presence of 2:1 A-V block. This is caused by retrograde concealed conduction in the A-V junction from the ventricular premature focus, resulting in a blocked P wave during the subsequent beat.
6. On the other hand, 3:1 A-V block may result when the atrial rate in 2:1 A-V block is enhanced by exercise or certain drugs. This is observed because the impaired A-V junctional tissue may respond only to every third atrial beat because of an abnormally prolonged refractory period.
7. For a similar reason, 4:1 A-V block may be due to actual 2:1 A-V block with concealed A-V conduction occurring at every fourth beat in Mobitz type II A-V block as well as in Mobitz type I A-V block.
8. From the above observations it can be seen that higher degree A-V block (i.e., 5:1, 6:1, 7:1, 8:1 A-V conduction) may actually be caused by a lesser degree A-V block (Mobitz type I or II) with concealed A-V conduction of varying degree.
9. As in second degree A-V block, BBBB may produce high degree A-V block. In this circumstance, BBBB is considered to be present when RBBB or LBBB is associated with high degree A-V block or when ventricular escape beats or rhythm are present to control the ventricular activity.

Clinical Significance

The clinical significance of high degree A-V block is very similar to that of complete A-V block and is discussed later in the chapter.

COMPLETE (THIRD DEGREE) A-V BLOCK

Complete (third degree) A-V block is characterized by independent atrial and ventricular activities resulting from complete block at the A-V junctional tissues, A-V (common) bundle, and bilateral bundle branches. When atrial impulses fail to conduct to the ventricles because of complete A-V block, a subsidiary pacemaker located anywhere distal to the site of block takes over ventricular activation. Among the many potential pacemakers located below the site of the block, the pacemaker with the fastest inherent rate takes over control of ventricular activity. In general, the A-V node acts as a pacemaker when the block occurs in the A-V junction, and the block in this case is usually caused by drug toxicity (i.e., DI), vagal influence, or acute diaphragmatic MI. In contrast, a pacemaker located in the A-V (common) bundle, bundle branches, or ventricles often takes over ventricular activity when the block is organic in nature (infranodal block).

In complete A-V block, the atrial rate is usually faster than the ventricular rate. Because of the independence of atrial and ventricular activities in complete A-V block, complete A-V dissociation always occurs. Complete A-V block is one of the three major basic rhythm disturbances responsible for the production of A-V dissociation.

Complete A-V block is a result of prolongation of the absolute refractory period so that it occupies the entire cardiac cycle. As a result, no relative refractory phase is present. Complete A-V block may be observed in various organic heart diseases, but the most common cause of complete A-V block is coronary artery disease (CAD). The next most common cause is DI. His bundle analysis of complete A-V block as well as the clinical significance of A-V nodal block versus infranodal block are summarized in Tables 2-2 and 2-4.

Diagnostic Criteria

The ECG findings of complete A-V block are summarized in Table 2-5.

TABLE 2-4. Complete A-V Block: Clinical Significance

Parameter	A-V Nodal Block	Infranodal Block
Disease process	A-V node	His-Purkinje system
Nature	Congenital or acquired	Always acquired
Age	Any age	Older than 45 years
Duration	Congenital: permanent Acquired: transient	Usually permanent
Damage to conduction tissue	Congenital: irreversible Acquired: reversible	Usually irreversible
Causes	Congenital: unknown Acquired: digitalis intoxication, diaphragmatic myocardial infarction, myocarditis, postcardiac operation	Chronic: unknown (degenerative-sclerotic?) Acute: acute anterior myocardial infarction
Symptoms	Often asymptomatic	Usually symptomatic

TABLE 2-5. Complete A-V Block: ECG Findings

Parameter	A-V Nodal Block	Infranodal Block
Site of block	A-V node	Three fascicles or His bundle
QRS contour of escape beats	Almost always normal Rarely abnormal (bundle branch block or hemiblock)	Always abnormal (broad)
Escape rate	45–60 beats/min	25–40 beats/min
Origin of escape beats	Lower A-V node (N-H region) or His bundle	Ventricles
Escape rhythm cycle	Regular	May be irregular and unstable

Relationship Between Atrial and Ventricular Activities

In complete (third degree) A-V block, atrial and ventricular activities must be unrelated throughout the tracing because of the complete blocking of the atrial impulses at the A-V junction, A-V (common) bundle, or bilateral bundle branches (Figure 2-6). By definition, complete A-V block cannot be diagnosed even if there is only a single ventricular captured beat. In complete A-V block, the atrial rate is always faster than the ventricular rate. The fact that complete A-V block is one of the three major underlying rhythm disorders producing A-V dissociation has been repeatedly emphasized.

Atrial Mechanism

The atria may be controlled by the sinus node (Figure 2-6A and B), or they may be controlled by any ectopic focus in the atria. Thus ectopic atrial mechanisms may include atrial fibrillation or flutter, or tachycardia. Very rarely, the atria and ventricles may be independently controlled by two pacemakers in the A-V junction to produce double A-V junctional rhythm. In this case, the atrial rate is, of course, faster than the ventricular rate. Double A-V junctional rhythm is one of the rarer causes of A-V dissociation.

Ventricular Mechanism

1. As none of the atrial impulses reaches the ventricles because of a block at the site mentioned before, A-V junctional escape rhythm or, less commonly, ventricular escape (idioventricular) rhythm develops to control the ventricles as a physiological mechanism.

2. When the subsidiary pacemaker is located above the bifurcation of the common bundle and in the A-V junctional tissue below the blocked zone, the QRS complex is usually normal in configuration (Figure 2-6). This type of ectopic rhythm is termed A-V junctional escape rhythm. In general, the ventricular rate in A-V junctional escape rhythm is between 40 and 60 beats/min (Figure 2-6), but it may be slower than 40 beats/min. In the latter case, an ectopic pacemaker is assumed to be located in the common bundle.

3. Aberrant ventricular conduction may occur in A-V junctional escape beats or rhythm. However, the escape beats or rhythm with slightly bizarre QRS configuration which was previously interpreted as "A-V

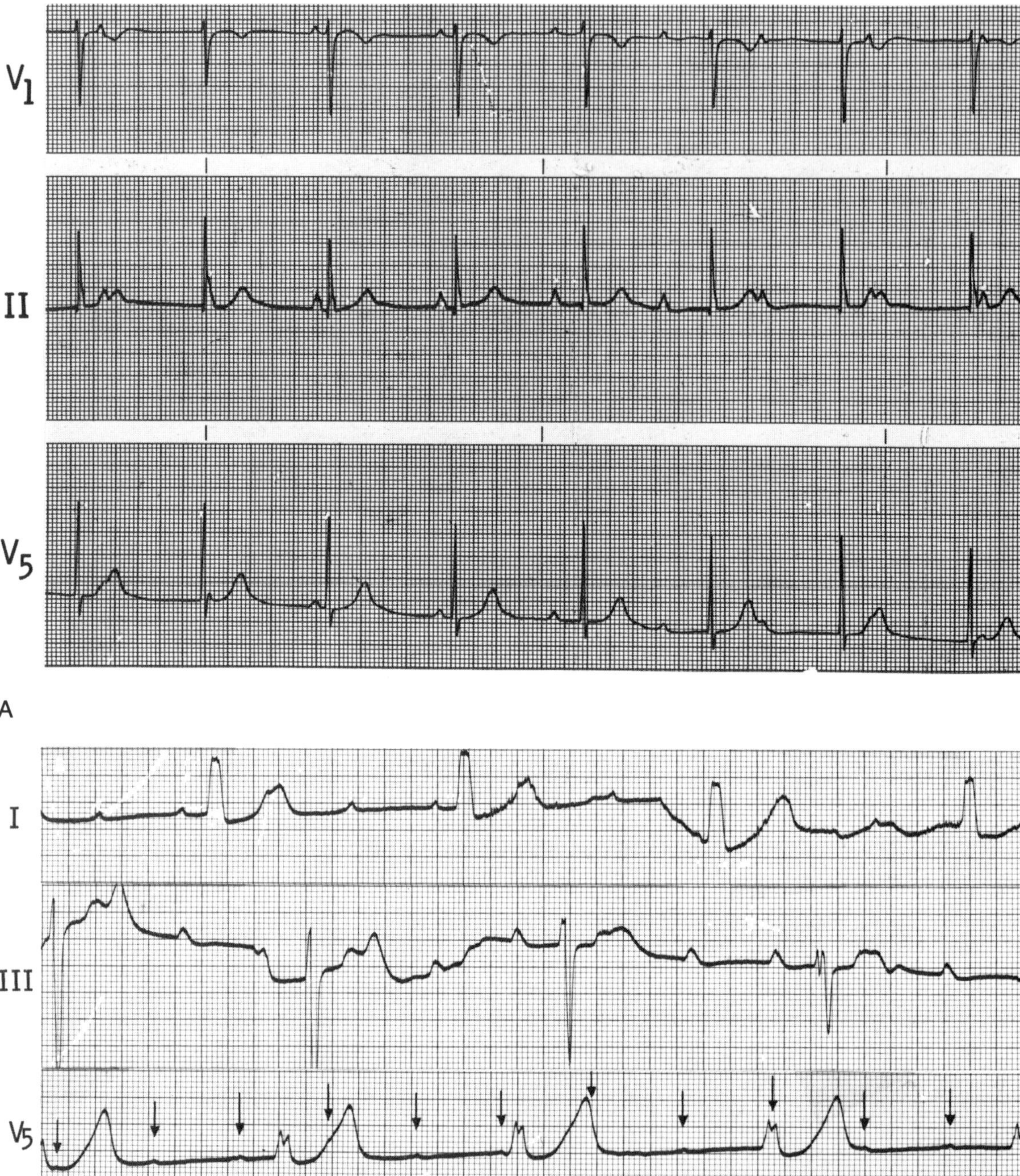

FIGURE 2-6. A: Sinus rhythm with A-V junctional escape rhythm due to complete A-V block (A-V nodal block). **B:** Sinus rhythm (*arrows*) with ventricular escape rhythm due to complete A-V block (infranodal block).

junctional escape beats or rhythm with aberrant ventricular conduction'' is now considered to be fascicular escape beats or rhythm in many cases. In addition, most of the escape rhythm with bizarre QRS complexes represents ventricular escape rhythm (Figure 2-6).

4. When the ectopic pacemaker is located below the bifurcation of the A-V (common) bundle, the configuration of the QRS complex is wide and bizarre because the propagation of the impulses in the ventricles occurs in an abnormal fashion (Figure 2-6). This type of ectopic rhythm is termed ventricular escape (idioventricular) rhythm, and its usual rate is between 30 and 40 beats/min. Occasionally, the ventricular rate is slower than 30 beats/min—sometimes as slow as 15 to 20 beats/min, particularly in elderly individuals.

5. Complete A-V block caused by a block within the His bundle was reported recently.

P-P and R-R Intervals

1. When the atrial mechanism is sinus, the P-P intervals are often regular, unless ordinary sinus arrhythmia or intermittent sinoatrial block is present.

2. In approximately 30% of cases of complete A-V block, the P-P interval which contains the QRS complex is shorter than the P-P interval without the QRS complex in spite of the independence of the atrial and ventricular activities. This is termed ventriculophasic sinus arrhythmia. Very rarely, the reverse phenomenon occurs.

3. The R-R intervals in A-V junctional or ventricular escape rhythm are usually regular.

4. However, not uncommonly, the R-R intervals in complete A-V block are irregular for various reasons, including:

1. Multiple pacemakers in the A-V junction and/or in the ventricles
2. Irregular discharge of a single pacemaker in the A-V junction or ventricles
3. Premature contractions (ventricular or A-V junctional)
4. Parasystole (ventricular or A-V junctional)
5. Exit block of varying degrees
6. Intermittent artificial pacemaker-induced ventricular rhythm

5. Of these, the commonest cause of irregular ventricular rhythm is an alteration in the rate of discharge from two or more pacemakers, particularly when the pacemakers are located in the ventricles.

6. Less commonly, two pacemakers may be located in the A-V junction. In these cases, one pacemaker gradually fades out periodically so that the other can take over with a different rate of discharge.

7. On the other hand, the rates of the ventricular escape rhythm may vary because of the irregular discharge of impulses from a single idioventricular pacemaker.

8. Rarely, more than two pacemakers in the A-V junction and/or ventricles produce multiple escape rhythms alternately or periodically.

9. The R-R intervals naturally become irregular in complete A-V block when premature contractions or parasystole of A-V junctional or ventricular origin coexist or when intermittent tachyarrhythmia occurs—leading to bradytachyarrhythmia syndrome.

10. In addition, exit block of varying degrees in A-V junctional or ventricular escape rhythm produces irregular ventricular cycles.

A-V Dissociation

As repeatedly emphasized, complete A-V block is one of the commonest causes of complete A-V dissociation.

Mechanism

1. Complete A-V block is commonly caused by a block at the A-V junction, and not uncommonly by a block at the A-V (common) bundle or bilateral bundle branches.

2. Depending on the etiological factors, complete A-V block may be transient or permanent.

3. For instance, complete A-V block resulting from acute diaphragmatic MI, DI, or acute myocarditis is usually transient, whereas anterior MI often produces a permanent complete A-V block (Table 2-4).

4. In addition, A-V junctional escape rhythm is almost always produced in transient complete A-V block because of reversible changes which occur at the A-V junction.

5. In contrast, ventricular escape rhythm is often produced in permanent complete A-V block because of irreversible damage below the bifurcation of the A-V bundle.

6. Chronic degenerative change in the A-V conduction system in elderly individuals likewise produces a permanent complete A-V block.

7. It has been shown that approximately 30 to 40% of all cases of complete A-V block are actually caused by BBBB.

8. Complete A-V block may result from a block within the His bundle.

9. Recently, paroxysmal complete A-V block has been considered to be related to phase 4 BBBB.

10. Bradycardia-dependent A-V block also has been reported.

11. In complete A-V block, the absolute refractory period is maximally prolonged in the A-V conduction system and occupies the entire cardiac cycle, leaving no time for a relative refractory period.

12. It is interesting to note that complete A-V block may be unidirectional, particularly in the A-V junction. That is, complete antegrade A-V block may exist in the presence of unimpaired retrograde ventriculoatrial conduction or vice versa. Thus it is not uncommon to observe one or more atrial captured beats in the presence of complete antegrade A-V block. Furthermore, artificial pacemaker-induced ventricular rhythm with occasional or even continuous atrial captured beats is not uncommon in spite of the fact that the artificial pacemaker was used for the treatment of complete A-V block.

Clinical Significance

Table 2-4 summarizes the clinical significance of complete A-V block.

1. The various factors responsible for the production of first, second, and high degree A-V block, described previously in this chapter, may also induce complete A-V block where the severity of the various causes is far advanced.

2. These factors include intoxication by various drugs (e.g., digitalis), acute infection (rheumatic fever, diphtheria, and various viral, bacterial, and fungal infections), electrolyte imbalances, trauma, cardiac surgery, CAD, etc. Complete A-V block produced by these conditions is often transient.

3. For example, complete A-V block of acute onset, which is most commonly caused by acute diaphragmatic MI or DI, is often transient because the damage in the A-V junction is usually reversible.

4. On the other hand, complete A-V block caused by an anterior MI is frequently permanent because of irreversible damage in the common bundle and/or both bundle branches.

5. Chronic acquired complete A-V block is most commonly caused by a degenerative process in the A-V conduction systems, especially in elderly individuals. In this population, chronic complete A-V block is often preceded by various ECG manifestations of incomplete BBBB (bifascicular or trifascicular block).

6. Less commonly, chronic acquired complete A-V block is caused by a chronic inflammatory process, e.g., rheumatic heart disease, diphtheria, syphilitic heart disease, or Chagas' heart disease.

7. Rarely, tumors or a granulomatous lesion (e.g., sarcoidosis), rheumatoid disease, and various cardiomyopathies produce complete A-V block.

8. In addition, permanent complete A-V block is occasionally induced by cardiac surgery.

9. Congenital complete A-V block may or may not be associated with other congenital cardiac anomalies. Common cardiac anomalies associated with congenital complete A-V block include Ebstein's disease and ventricular septal defect.

10. Familial complete A-V block has been reported.

11. Various symptoms and signs may be observed in complete A-V block.

Symptoms and Signs

1. Needless to say, various symptoms and signs resulting from the underlying heart disease and CHF are observed.

2. In general, the symptoms in complete A-V block are markedly different in the congenital and the acquired forms.

3. Congenital complete A-V block without other cardiac anomalies is usually asymptomatic.

4. Conversely, acquired complete A-V block nearly always produces various symptoms.

5. This discrepancy is attributed to a higher incidence of advanced heart disease in older people with acquired complete A-V block compared to those with the congenital form.

6. In addition, various symptoms in complete A-V block are greatly influenced by the ventricular rate and the underlying causes, especially the severity of the heart disease.

7. When the ventricular mechanism is A-V junctional escape rhythm, complete A-V block per se may not produce any symptoms because of

a relatively rapid ventricular rate in addition to normal intraventricular conduction.

8. In congenital complete A-V block, an A-V junctional escape rhythm is nearly always present because the block occurs above the bifurcation of the A-V (common) bundle.

9. On the other hand, severe CHF and Adams-Stokes syndrome frequently occur in patients with acquired complete A-V block, particularly when the ventricular rate is slow (ventricular escape rhythm) and advanced heart disease exists. This is because the cardiac output is further reduced when the ventricular mechanism is ventricular escape (idioventricular) rhythm as the ventricles are activated in an abnormal fashion in addition to the markedly slow ventricular rate.

Treatment

The therapeutic approach depends on various factors, particularly the underlying disease process, the site of complete A-V block, the ventricular rate, and the presence or absence of symptoms. All complete infranodal blocks (complete trifascicular block) (Figure 2-6B) must receive permanent artificial pacemaker implantation (see Chapters 3 and 8). Complete intranodal block (A-V nodal block), as is seen in acute diaphragmatic MI or DI, may not require active treatment so long as the ventricular rate is relatively fast (more than 45 beats/min) and the patient is asymptomatic.

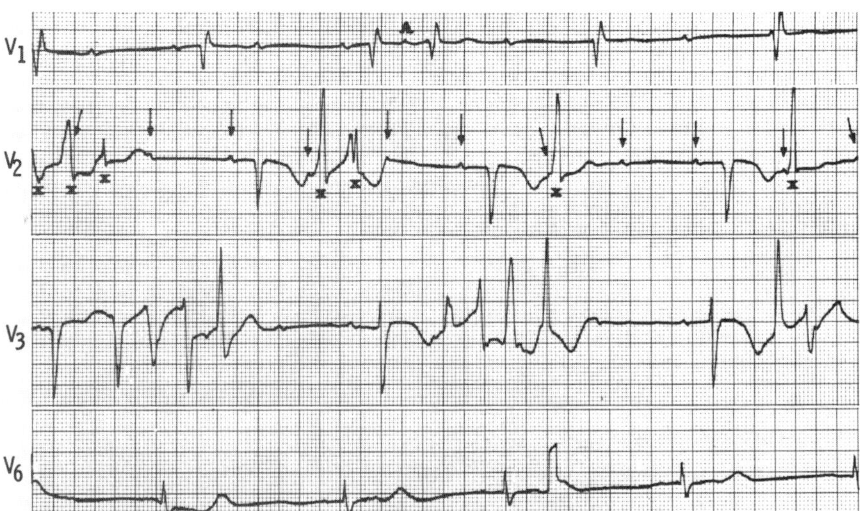

FIGURE 2-7. Figures 2-7 and 2-8 were obtained from the same patient, who had an acute anteroseptal MI. In Figure 2-7 the *arrows* indicate P waves. The tracing shows sinus rhythm (atrial rate: 75 beats/min) with 2:1 A-V block with intermittent high degree A-V block and frequent VPCs (*X*) with group beats. These ECG findings represent brady-tachyarrhythmia syndrome. In addition, there is RBBB.

Prognosis

The prognosis in complete A-V block depends largely on the cause, the presence or absence and the severity of the underlying heart disease, whether CHF exists, and the response to therapy. Transient complete A-V block may disappear completely within 1 to 2 weeks when the underlying cause (e.g., acute diaphragmatic MI or DI) is well treated. It has been shown that many patients with congenital complete A-V block often have a normal life expectancy unless a significant congenital cardiac anomaly coexists. In addition, many elderly patients with chronic complete A-V block are able to carry on productive lives for many years because various types of artificial pacemaker are readily available. However, the mortality rate is extremely high in patients with complete A-V block (complete trifascicular block) caused by acute anterior MI, even after artificial pacing, because of many other complications, including cardiogenic shock and congestive heart failure.

BRADYTACHYARRHYTHMIA SYNDROME

The term bradytachyarrhythmia syndrome is used when the cardiac rhythm disorder consists of a bradyarrhythmia component and a tachyarrhythmia component. The fact that bradytachyarrhythmia syndrome is frequently a late manifestation of SSS is stressed in Chapter 4. On the other hand, bradytachyarrhythmia syndrome may occur in the absence of SSS. Under this circumstance the bradyarrhythmia component is commonly advanced, or complete A-V block, whereas the tachyarrhythmia component is frequently VPCs, ventricular group beats, and ventricular tachycardia (Figure 2-7). Antiarrhythmic drug therapy alone is usually unsatisfactory for the treatment of bradytachyarrhythmia syndrome. Most patients require artificial cardiac pacing (Figure 2-8). In addition, one or more antiarrhythmic agents—e.g., quinidine, diisopyramide phosphate (Norpace), procainamide—may be necessary when the tachyarrhythmia component is not suppressed by artificial cardiac pacing. On the other hand, in many cases overdrive pacing (rate: 80 to 120 beats/min) is effective in the control of both bradyarrhythmia and tachyarrhythmia components.

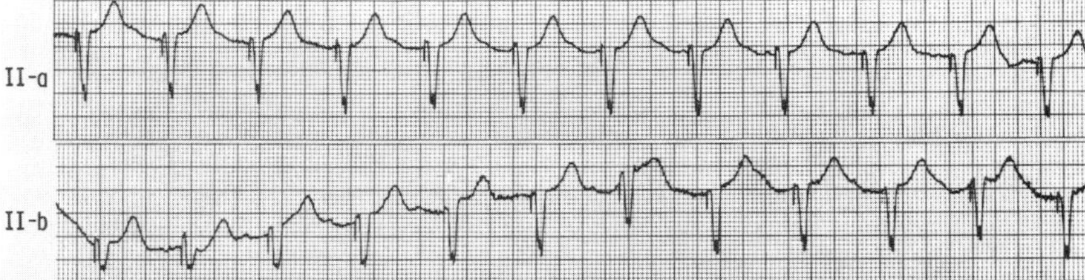

FIGURE 2-8. Leads II-a and II-b are continuous. An artificial pacemaker with a slight overdriving pacing rate (rate: 80 beats/min) was effective for the bradytachyarrhythmia syndrome shown in Figure 2-7.

Intraventricular Conduction Disturbances

3

Various intraventricular conduction disturbances may occur in various clinical circumstances. The most common and well recognized intraventricular conduction disturbances are right and left bundle branch block (RBBB and LBBB). In bundle branch block, the impulse is conducted via an intact bundle branch so that the ventricle with a blocked bundle branch is activated later than the ventricle with the intact bundle branch. Therefore, instead of simultaneous activation of both ventricles under normal circumstances, bundle branch block produces asynchronous activation of the two ventricles. The incidence of LBBB and RBBB is considered to be almost equal.

Although less well recognized, some intraventricular conduction disturbances are caused by a conduction delay that involves both ventricles diffusely. This type of delay, termed nonspecific or diffuse intraventricular conduction disturbance, is seen, for example, in advanced hyperkalemia or procainamide toxicity. As a rule, intraventricular conduction disturbances are recognized by a prolongation of the QRS interval, although some of these disturbances produce little or no prolongation of the QRS interval. For example, a block at one of the subdivisions of the left bundle branch system (hemiblock) causes an abnormal QRS axis deviation without significant alteration in the QRS interval.

Bundle branch block has been reported in healthy individuals, but it has a close relationship to ventricular hypertrophy. This is more often true for LBBB because the underlying process of LBBB is commonly left ventricular hypertrophy, particularly in adults. Various intraventricular conduction disturbances are frequently produced as a result of permanent damage to the conduction system from acute anterior myocardial infarction (MI). In addition, some cardiac lesions, e.g., an atrial septal defect, are almost always associated with RBBB *pattern*. RBBB or LBBB, hemiblocks, and bifascicular (BFB) and trifascicular (TFB) blocks are also common after cardiac surgery, particularly in various congenital heart diseases. Familial bundle branch block and bifascicular or trifascicular block have been reported.

When the conduction disturbances involve both right and left bundle branches and/or one of the fascicles of the left bundle branch system, various ECG abnormalities are produced. This situation is termed bilateral bundle branch block (BBBB). BBBB includes bifascicular and trifascicular blocks, and in many cases BBBB is incomplete. Complete A-V block is produced when the block in both bundle branches is complete or RBBB and both fascicles of the left bundle branch are blocked simultaneously (complete trifascicular block).

It is essential to understand the concept of hemiblocks and bifascicular and trifascicular blocks fully in order to understand certain atrioventricular (A-V) conduction disturbances in depth (see Chapter 2). For example, Mobitz type II A-V block (see Figure 2-2) is considered to be a precursor of complete A-V block (infranodal block) resulting from complete trifascicular block. For the same reason, the site of the Mobitz type II A-V block is in the infranodal region. In addition, Mobitz type II A-V block is almost always associated with LBBB, RBBB, or bifascicular block. Clinically, therefore, permanent artificial pacemaker implantation is recommended for every patient with Mobitz type II A-V block regardless of whether the patient is symptomatic (see Chapter 8). Moreover, prophylactic artificial pacing is recommended for all patients who develop BFB or TFB as a result of acute anterior myocardial infarction (see Chapter 7). Various manifestations of BBBB (both bifascicular and trifascicular blocks) are summarized in Table 3-1. Hemiblocks and BBBB are discussed in detail in this chapter.

HEMIBLOCKS

The left bundle branch consists of two subdivisions: anterior (superior) and posterior (inferior). The anterior division of the left bundle branch traverses the base of the anterior papillary muscle of the left ventricle, whereas the posterior division runs toward the posterior papillary muscle. Anatomically, the anterior division is located superiorly and the posterior division inferiorly (Figure 3-1). When these two subdivisions are intact, the impulse is transmitted to the left ventricle via the anterior and posterior divisions simultaneously (Figure 3-1A).

TABLE 3-1. Diagnostic Criteria of Bilateral Bundle Branch Block

1. Right bundle branch block with left anterior hemiblock
2. Right bundle branch block with left posterior hemiblock
3. Alternating left and right bundle branch block
4. Left or right bundle branch block with first or second degree A-V block (infranodal block)
5. Left or right bundle branch block with prolonged H-V interval > 55 msec
6. Left bundle branch block on one occasion and right bundle branch block on another
7. Mobitz type II A-V block
8. Any combination of the above findings
9. Complete A-V block with ventricular escape (idioventricular) rhythm

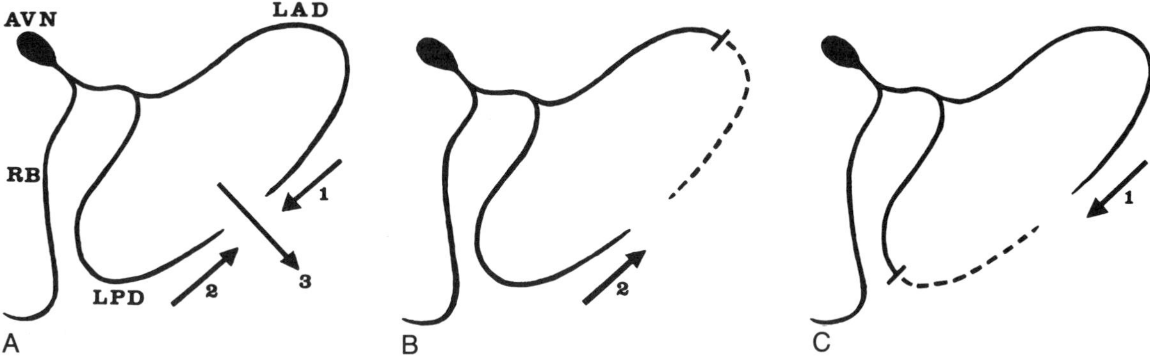

FIGURE 3-1. Hemiblocks. When both anterior and posterior divisions of the left bundle branch system are intact **(A),** the left ventricle is activated via both divisions (vectors 1 and 2) so that the resultant forces of vectors 1 and 2 produce vector 3. However, when one of two divisions of the left bundle branch system is blocked, the impulses must travel through the intact division only. That is, in anterior hemiblock **(B)** vector 1 is no longer present, and as a result the left ventricle is activated via the intact posterior division (vector 2). In this case the electrical axis shifts to the left and superiorly (left axis deviation). For the same reason, posterior hemiblock **(C)** produces right axis deviation because the left ventricle is activated via the intact anterior division (vector 1). (*RB*) right bundle branch. (*AVN*) A-V node. (*LAD*) left anterior division. (*LPD*) left posterior division.

Diagnostic Criteria

The term "hemiblock" is used when one of the subdivisions of the left bundle branch system is blocked.

1. In left anterior (superior) hemiblock, the impulse is transmitted through the intact posterior division to activate the left ventricle.
2. Because the impulse conducted via the posterior division is directed superiorly and to the left (Figure 3-1B), marked left axis deviation is observed in left anterior hemiblock.
3. In addition, a small q wave in lead I with a small r wave in lead III is usually observed in left anterior hemiblock because of downward and rightward initial septal activation.
4. The above findings are observed in left anterior hemiblock specifically because the posterior papillary muscle is located not only inferiorly but also medial to the anterior papillary muscle.
5. After septal activation, major ventricular forces are directed superiorly and to the left, leading to marked left axis deviation (more than −45 degrees) in left anterior hemiblock.
6. Conversely, in left posterior hemiblock the left ventricle is activated via an intact anterior division.
7. Because the impulse conducted through the anterior division is

directed inferiorly and to the right, right axis deviation is produced in left posterior hemiblock (Figure 3-1C).

8. A small r wave in lead I with a small q wave in lead III is observed in left posterior hemiblock because the initial vector is directed superiorly and to the left.

9. There is usually little (0.01 to 0.02 sec) or no prolongation of the QRS interval in hemiblocks because the Purkinje fibers in areas of the left anterior and posterior divisions are richly confluent.

10. In other words, marked left axis deviation and right axis deviation are manifestations of left anterior and posterior hemiblock, respectively.

11. Hemiblocks may occur intermittently, which is analogous to intermittent bundle branch block.

12. However, it should be pointed out that abnormal QRS axis deviation is not necessarily caused by hemiblocks. For example, right axis deviation is commonly a result of right ventricular hypertrophy or acute pulmonary embolism.

13. The diagnostic criteria of *left anterior hemiblock* are:

1. Marked left axis deviation (−45 to −90 degrees)
2. Small q waves in lead I and a small r wave in lead III
3. Little or no prolongation of the QRS interval
4. No evidence of other factors responsible for left axis deviation (true or pseudo)

14. The diagnostic criteria of *left posterior hemiblock* are:

1. Marked right axis deviation (+105 to +180 degrees)
2. A small r wave in lead I and a small q wave in lead III
3. Little or no prolongation of the QRS interval
4. No evidence of other factors responsible for right axis deviation (true or pseudo)

A pure form of hemiblock is not uncommon, especially during acute anterior myocardial infarction, but RBBB often coexists with hemiblock (see Figure 2-5). A pure form of left anterior hemiblock is much more common than left posterior hemiblock. Left posterior hemiblock frequently coexists with RBBB to produce BFB as a manifestation of incomplete BBBB (Figure 3-2). Why the incidence of left posterior hemiblock is much lower than that of left anterior hemiblock can be explained as follows: The posterior division is shorter and thicker, and is less influenced by stresses of outflow pressure because of its inflow tract structure. In addition, it has a double blood supply compared to that of the left anterior division.

Clinical Significance

Hemiblock is one of the most common ECG abnormalities in our practice.

1. Many elderly individuals with no clinical evidence of organic heart disease may have left anterior hemiblock.

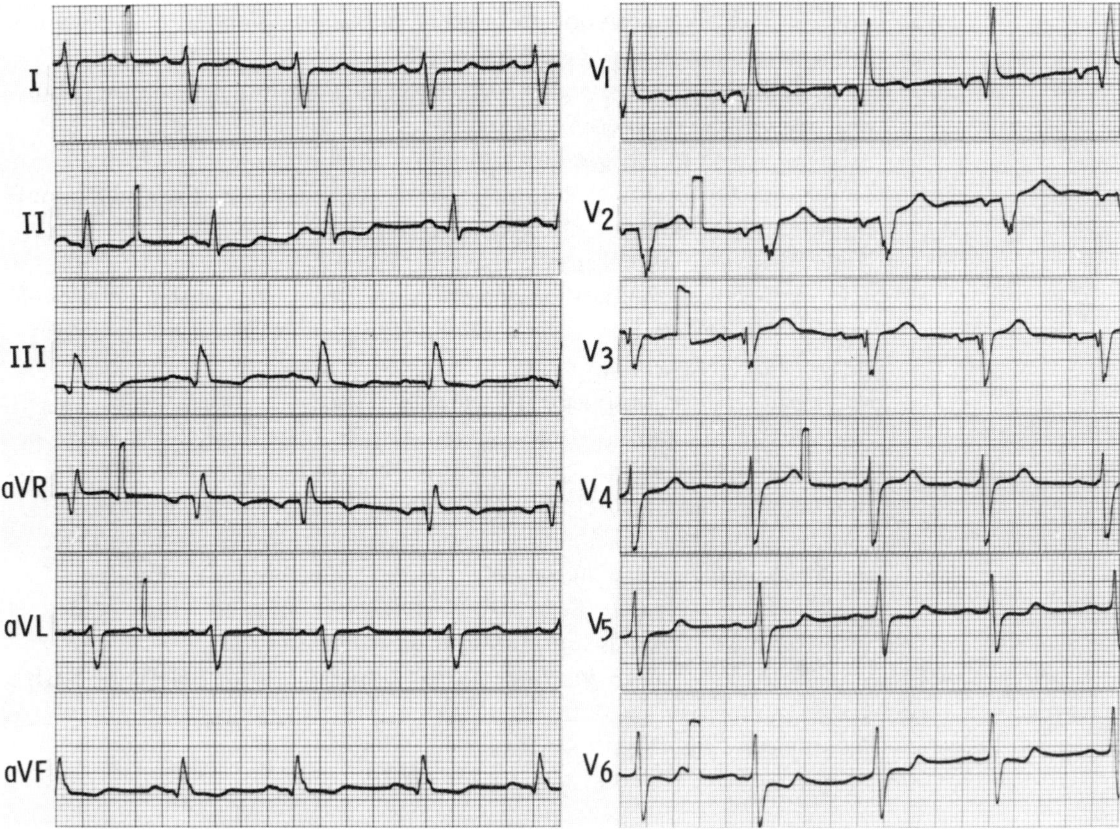

FIGURE 3-2. BFB consisting of RBBB and left posterior hemiblock due to a recent anteroseptal MI. The rhythm is sinus. Old diaphragmatic MI is also a possibility.

2. Isolated left posterior hemiblock is much less common.
3. The most common underlying disease in individuals with hemiblocks, e.g., LBBB, is hypertensive heart disease.
4. Hemiblocks with acute onset are nearly always caused by acute anterior MI.
5. Less commonly, hemiblocks are encountered in cardiomyopathies and calcific aortic stenosis.
6. In addition, hemiblocks may be found in myocarditis, during coronary arteriograpy, or in the postoperative period following cardiac surgery.
7. Hemiblocks may be observed in association with hyperkalemia.
8. Recently, a transient hemiblock was observed after physical exercise.

BIFASCICULAR AND TRIFASCICULAR BLOCK

Diagnostic Criteria

The term bifascicular block is used when two fascicles are blocked simultaneously. Bifascicular block is a form of incomplete BBBB (Table 3-1).

1. The most common form of BFB is a combination of RBBB and left anterior hemiblock (see Figure 2-5).

2. BFB consisting of RBBB and left posterior hemiblock (Figure 3-2) occurs rather uncommonly.

3. The term trifascicular block is used specifically when a block simultaneously involves the three peripheral fascicles: the right bundle branch and the anterior and posterior divisions of the left bundle branch. Thus TFB is an expression of BBBB (Table 3-1).

4. When all three of the peripheral fascicles are completely blocked, needless to say complete A-V block (complete TFB) is the end result. In this case, ventricular escape (idioventricular) rhythm with a very slow ventricular rate is produced (see Figure 2-6).

5. The diagnosis of incomplete TFB is certain when the same patient exhibits a combination of RBBB and left posterior hemiblock on one occasion and RBBB with left anterior hemiblock on another.

6. Various ECG manifestations are produced when one or more of the three fascicles are incompletely and/or intermittently blocked.

7. Extremely complicated ECG findings can result when the degree of incomplete block differs in the three fascicles.

8. A-V block of varying degree associated with RBBB or LBBB and/or anterior or posterior hemiblock is usually a typical example of incomplete TFB (Figure 3-3).

Clinical Significance and Therapeutic Approach

The clinical significance of BFB or TFB varies markedly depending on the onset and progress of the block.

1. For example, chronic BFB or incomplete TFB is often asymptomatic, and no particular treatment is indicated so long as the patient is asymptomatic.

2. On the other hand, prophylactic artificial pacing is required when the patient develops BFB or incomplete TFB acutely as a result of acute anterior MI (see Figure 2-5). An artificial pacemaker is recommended in this case regardless of symptoms because complete (infranodal) A-V block may soon follow.

3. Acute hemiblock, BFB, or TFB may be observed in patients with marked hyperkalemia and myocarditis.

4. These intraventricular conduction disturbances are also not uncommon during the postoperative period for various cardiac lesions and during cardiac catheterization.

5. Among congenital heart diseases, the atrial septal defect, ostium secundum type, is frequently associated with an RBBB *pattern* with normal or right axis deviation of the QRS complexes.

6. On the other hand, BFB consisting of RBBB and left anterior hemiblock is often observed in patients with atrial septal defect, ostium primum type.

7. Tetralogy of Fallot is commonly associated with RBBB and left posterior hemiblock, causing BFB. Under these circumstances, congen-

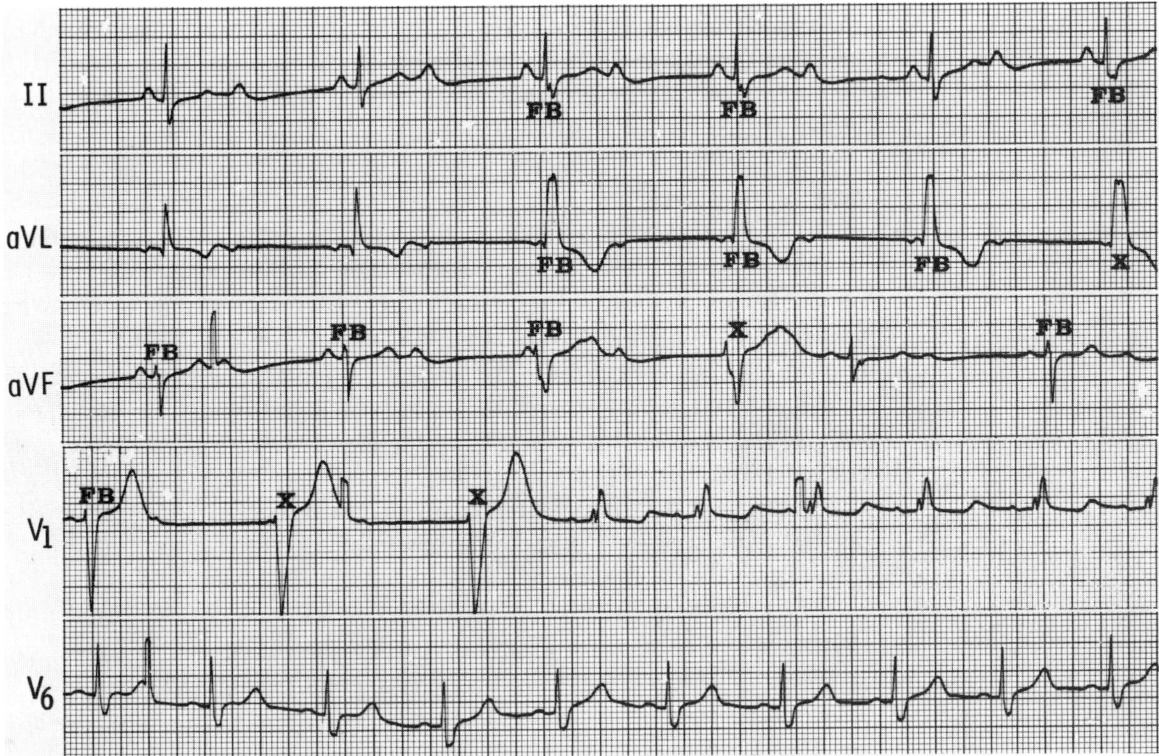

FIGURE 3-3. Sinus rhythm with intermittent 2:1 A-V block and RBBB. In addition, there are areas showing ventricular escape rhythm (*X*) caused by advanced A-V block. Note the frequent ventricular fusion beats (*FB*). These ECG findings represent advanced but incomplete TFB.

ital BFB does not seem to progress to a higher degree BBBB. Therefore an artificial pacemaker is *not* indicated.

8. Chronic BFB or incomplete TFB may lead to complete A-V block sometime in the future, but it is impossible to predict the exact time when complete (infranodal) A-V block will be produced.

9. Two major factors primarily determine the indications for permanent artificial cardiac pacing. The first and most important factor is the presence of symptoms (e.g., dizziness, near-syncope, syncope) due directly to a slow ventricular rate (usually less than 45 beats/min). Needless to say, permanent artificial pacing is urgently needed for patients with complete A-V block caused by complete TFB leading to very slow ventricular escape rhythm (see Figure 2-6). The second factor is the ventricular rate itself. When this rate is slower than 45 beats/min in patients with chronic BFB or TFB, permanent artificial pacing is indicated even if the patient is asymptomatic.

10. Permanent pacing is also indicated when advanced BBBB is associated with frequent ventricular premature contractions (VPCs) or ectopic tachyarrhythmia causing bradytachyarrhythmia syndrome.

11. Mobitz type II A-V block is an expression of incomplete BBBB

(incomplete infranodal block; see Chapter 2) for which permanent cardiac pacing is mandatory (see Figure 2-2).

12. When 2:1 A-V block is associated with bundle branch block (either left or right) or BFB, it is considered to be a variant of Mobitz type II A-V block. Permanent cardiac pacing is definitely indicated in these cases (see Figure 2-3).

13. When BBBB is further advanced, complex rhythm abnormalities are produced. For example, advanced incomplete BBBB may be manifested by RBBB or LBBB with 2:1 or Mobitz type II A-V block, with areas of complete A-V block as a result of complete TFB producing a ventricular escape rhythm (Figure 3-3). Another example is advanced A-V block of varying degree (e.g., 3:1 or 4:1 A-V block) associated with RBBB or LBBB (or alternating bundle branch block) and intermittent complete A-V block.

14. Eventually, advanced incomplete BBBB leads to complete BBBB, causing complete A-V block as a result of complete TFB (see Figure 2-6).

15. Prophylactic pacing has been generally recommended for all patients who demonstrate RBBB or LBBB associated with a prolonged H-V interval (the interval from the His bundle potential to the ventricular potential) on the His bundle ECG even in asymptomatic individuals, but this view is not accepted uniformly.

4 Sick Sinus Syndrome

There has been an increasing awareness of the clinical entity the ''sick sinus syndrome (SSS)'' during the past decade. The syndrome is found to be relatively common in our practice, particularly among elderly individuals, and it can be successfully treated with artificial cardiac pacing in most cases. The term SSS has been used to describe a broad spectrum of clinical manifestations—e.g., syncope or near-syncope, dizziness, increased congestive heart failure (CHF), and/or angina and palpitations—as a result of a dysfunctioning sinus node. Electrocardiographic (ECG) manifestations in SSS may include: (1) persistent and marked sinus bradycardia; (2) sinoatrial (S-A) block; (3) sinus arrest; (4) a long pause after an atrial premature contraction (APC); (5) chronic atrial fibrillation or atrial flutter with slow ventricular rate; (6) carotid sinus hypersensitivity; (7) no stable sinus rhythm after cardioversion; (8) atrioventricular (A-V) junctional escape rhythm with or without slow and unstable sinus activity; and (9) bradytachyarrhythmia syndrome (BTS). These ECG findings in SSS are *not* drug-induced.

Various terms have been used to describe these phenomena, including sick sinus syndrome, sinoatrial syncope, sluggish sinus node syndrome, inadequate sinus mechanism, sick sinus node, and lazy sinus node. When tachyarrhythmia components are present intermittently or periodically during slow rhythm, various terms have been used, e.g., bradytachyarrhythmia syndrome (BTS), bradytachy syndrome, and tachycardia-bradycardia syndrome. Although some investigators use the terms SSS and BTS interchangeably, BTS is one of the common manifestations of SSS in most cases.

As can be expected, the degree of sinus node dysfunction may be so minimal that the SSS manifests only by slight sinus bradycardia. In this case, the patient is usually asymptomatic. On the other hand, the sinus node may be severely diseased, leading to complete generator failure—prolonged sinus arrest or AF with slow ventricular rate. Advanced

SSS is nearly always symptomatic. Various symptoms in SSS are usually related to either cardiac or cerebral dysfunction: The perfusion deficit in these organs is responsible for the production of various symptoms in SSS. Syncope or near-syncope is the most common clinical manifestation of SSS.

ANATOMY AND ELECTROPHYSIOLOGY

1. The sinus node has both sympathetic and parasympathetic (vagal) innervation, but the latter is richer in the A-V node. The electrophysiological event spontaneous phase 4 depolarization is the determining factor that distinguishes between the pacemaker cells and all other cells in the body. The sinus node is the dominant pacemaker because the sinus node cells possess the fastest spontaneous depolarization. Spontaneous sinus node depolarization can be altered by parasympathetic and sympathetic influences: Vagal stimulation or acetylcholine can slow automaticity of the sinus node by reducing the slope of phase 4 depolarization as well as hyperpolarizing the cells. On the other hand, sympathetic stimulation or catecholamine infusion enhances the spontaneous sinus node discharge rate, primarily as a result of an increase in the rate of phase 4 depolarization.

2. Various investigative studies have confirmed that the sinus node is the primary pacemaker in the heart. Because the sinus node has a faster inherent rate than any other cardiac pacemaker, sinus rhythm is present in the majority of healthy individuals. In SSS, when the sinus node produces cardiac impulses that are slower than usual (sinus bradycardia) or fails to produce any impulse (sinus arrest), or the sinus impulse is not conducted to the atria because of S-A block, the subsidiary pacemaker (commonly the A-V junction) takes over the ventricular activity as an escape mechanism. On the other hand, chronic generator failure (sinus arrest) not uncommonly leads to the establishment of chronic atrial fibrillation (often with a slow ventricular rate).

3. The sinus node is approximately 15 mm in length, 5 to 7 mm in width, and 1.5 to 2.0 mm in thickness. Its shape varies, but by and large it resembles a snail extended from its shell, which misleads one to think of the node as having a head, a body, and a tail. Because the sinus node is situated less than 1 mm beneath the epicardial surface, it is vulnerable to many disease processes, including trauma (e.g., pericarditis). The superficial anatomical location of the sinus node is often directly or indirectly responsible for the development of SSS.

4. The sinus node artery in the human heart is commonly located near the center of the sinus node, although it may be sited eccentrically. In approximately 55 to 60% of human hearts, the sinus node artery arises from the proximal 2 to 3 cm of the right coronary artery, whereas in 40 to 45% of cases it arises from the proximal 1 cm of the left circumflex coronary artery. Other origins of the sinus node artery are rare, accounting for only about 2% of the total. At times there are two branches of the sinus node artery of equal size. The sinus node artery, regardless of

whether it arises from the right or left coronary artery, courses along the anteromedial atrial wall of the base of the superior vena cava, which it encircles. This artery anastomoses with other atrial arteries of both ipsilateral and contralateral origin. Generally, the primary arterial supply of the sinus node is unilateral in origin. Smaller branches of the artery are distributed throughout the sinus node, as are small veins; large veins are present infrequently.

5. Microscopically, the sinus node is composed of three types of cell: P cells, transitional cells, and working cells. The term P cell has been used because of the cell's pale appearance, resembling the primitive myocardial cell. P cells are thought to be responsible for sinus node pacemaker function.

6. The Purkinje-like fibers, the ''internodal pathways'' which connect the sinus node to the specialized atrial conduction tissue, have been described as the anterior, middle, and posterior internodal tracts. It has been demonstrated by electrophysiological studies that the cardiac impulse from the sinus node reaches the A-V node more rapidly than it would if it were conducted through the ordinary myocardium. Although any one of three internodal pathways may be responsible for intraatrial conduction, it is thought that in most normal hearts the conduction is carried out preferentially via the anterior tract. This view is not uniformly accepted, however.

UNDERLYING CAUSES

Although various drugs, e.g., digitalis, propranolol, and quinidine, frequently cause dysfunction of the sinus node, these functionally reversible effects on the sinus node are not considered part of the SSS. The basic underlying causes of SSS are anatomical, with physiological consequences which produce a longstanding and often irreversible process in the sinus node.

Coronary Artery Disease

1. Coronary artery disease (CAD), particularly myocardial infarction (MI), has been reported to be the most common underlying disease that produces SSS.

2. Dysfunction of the sinus node has been reported to occur in approximately 5% of patients with acute MI. In addition, sinus node dysfunction can be expected to be present in half of the patients with diaphragmatic MI.

3. Dysfunction of the sinus node is usually observed during the first 4 days of MI in this circumstance.

4. Commonly, sinus node dysfunction manifests as progressive sinus bradycardia followed by various supraventricular arrhythmias, including atrial fibrillation or flutter and A-V junctional escape rhythm with a periodic restoration of sinus bradycardia and intermittent sinus arrest or S-A block.

5. Atrial MI causes the sinus node dysfunction on rare occasions. Atrial damage, including sinus node dysfunction, very commonly results from main right coronary artery occlusion (causing diaphragmatic MI) and left circumflex artery occlusion (causing anterolateral MI).

Sclerotic-Degenerative Process

1. When one eliminates CAD as a cause of SSS, the majority of the remaining cases show no clear evidence of the clinical heart disease responsible for the production of the SSS. In this circumstance, sclerotic-degenerative process involving the sinus node is thought to be responsible for the SSS in most cases.

2. Histological studies revealed that severe fibrosis involving the sinus node and S-A junction was the main feature of SSS.

3. In some cases of SSS, amyloid infiltration involving the sinus node was demonstrated.

Other Disorders

Many other underlying causes may be responsible for producing SSS as well.

1. These include rheumatic heart disease (RHD), cardiomyopathies, congenital heart disease, surgical trauma, hypertension, pericarditis, myocarditis, amyloidosis, systemic lupus erythematosus, muscular dystrophy, Friedreich's ataxia, malignancy, hemochromatosis, and diphtheria.

2. A familial incidence of the SSS has been reported.

3. An association of SSS with long Q-T syndrome also has been described.

4. Recently, SSS associated with systemic embolism and mitral valve prolapse syndrome (MVPS) has been reported.

ECG MANIFESTATIONS

Depending on the degree of sinus node dysfunction, various ECG abnormalities may be produced in SSS (Table 4-1). Persisting and severe sinus bradycardia (not caused by drugs) is the most common (75 to 80% of all patients with SSS) and the earliest manifestation of SSS; other ECG abnormalities follow as the syndrome progresses. In longstanding SSS, AF is the commonest underlying rhythm. When SSS is far advanced, it manifests as bradytachyarrhythmia syndrome in which a variety of cardiac rhythms are observed in many cases. In addition, A-V conduction disturbances as well as intraventricular block often coexist in many patients with advanced SSS.

Sinus Bradycardia

Although some degree of sinus bradycardia is common in many healthy individuals, especially athletes, persistent and marked sinus bradycardia (not caused by various drugs) deserves medical investigation.

TABLE 4-1. Sick Sinus Syndrome: ECG Manifestations

1. Marked and persisting sinus bradycardia
2. Sinus arrest and/or S-A block
3. Drug (e.g., atropine, Isuprel) resistant sinus bradyarrhythmias
4. Long pause after an APC
5. Prolonged sinus node recovery time determined by atrial pacing
6. Chronic AF or repetitive occurrence of AF (less commonly atrial flutter):
   a. With slow ventricular rate
   b. Preceded or followed by sinus bradycardia, sinus arrest, or S-A block
7. A-V junctional escape rhythm (with or without slow and unstable sinus activity)
8. Carotid sinus syncope
9. Failure of restoration of sinus rhythm after cardioversion
10. Bradytachyarrhythmia syndrome
11. Common coexisting A-V block and/or intraventricular block
12. Any combination of the above

1. SSS should be strongly suspected when chronic sinus bradycardia shows a rate slower than 45 beats/min with or without symptoms.

2. Marked sinus bradycardia may produce symptoms, e.g., lightheadedness, near-syncope, or syncope.

3. It should be certain that sinus bradycardia is not caused by drugs, e.g., propranolol (Inderal), digitalis, reserpine (Serpasil), guanethidine (Ismelin), and methyldopa (Aldomet).

4. On the other hand, SSS may be unmasked by small amounts of drugs, particularly digitalis or propranolol. In other words, marked sinus bradycardia after administration of a small amount of these drugs strongly suggests the presence of SSS, especially in elderly individuals.

5. When sinus bradycardia is marked, one or more A-V junctional escape beats may occur and incomplete A-V dissociation is often produced (Figure 4-1). At times, marked sinus bradycardia leads to A-V junctional escape bigeminy in which sinus beats and A-V junctional escape beats occur on every other beat. When the A-V and sinus nodes are both diseased, a common occurrence, the A-V junctional escape rhythm also produces a markedly slow rate.

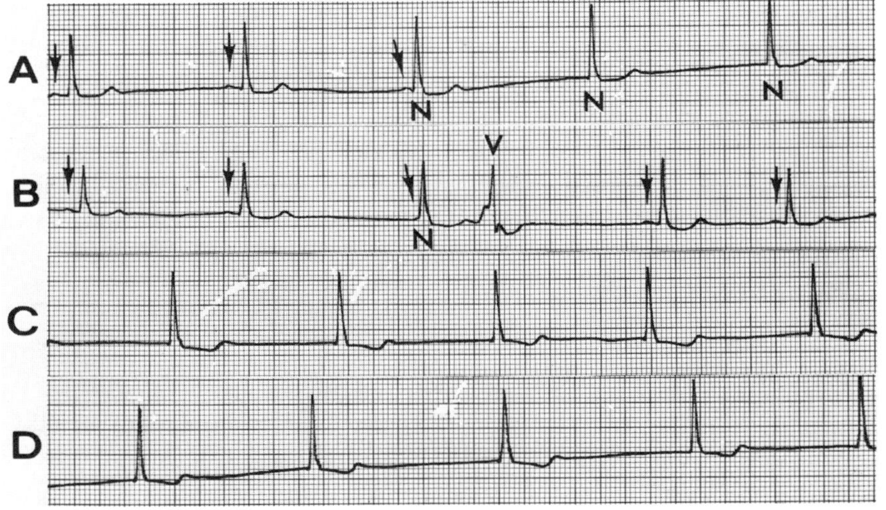

FIGURE 4-1. The Holter monitor ECG rhythm strips **A** to **D** are not continuous. The rhythm is sinus bradycardia (*arrows*) with intermittent A-V junctional escape rhythm (*N*) and occasional VPCs (*V*). These ECG findings represent an early manifestation of SSS.

6. At times ventricular escape beats seem to control the ventricular activity in severe sinus bradycardia when the A-V node is unable to produce the expected escape impulses because of permanent disease of the A-V node.

7. Marked sinus bradycardia is often irregular and may be followed by atrial or ventricular tachyarrhythmias leading to BTS (Figures 1-6, 4-2, and 4-3).

8. First degree A-V block (P-R interval of 0.24 sec or more) also commonly coexists.

Sinus Arrest and/or S-A Block

1. When SSS further progresses, the sinus node fails to produce any cardiac impulse leading to sinus arrest. The long P-P interval caused by sinus arrest has no relationship to the basic P-P cycle.

2. During sinus arrest it is common to observe one or more A-V junctional (less commonly ventricular) escape beats that control the ventricular activity.

3. S-A block may be observed in some patients with SSS. In those with S-A block the sinus impulse is unable to conduct to the atria as a result of a block at the S-A junction (Figure 4-4).

4. S-A block has two forms: Mobitz type I and II. Mobitz type II S-A block is characterized by an intermittent absence of the expected P wave(s) in which the long P-P interval is a multiple of the basic P-P

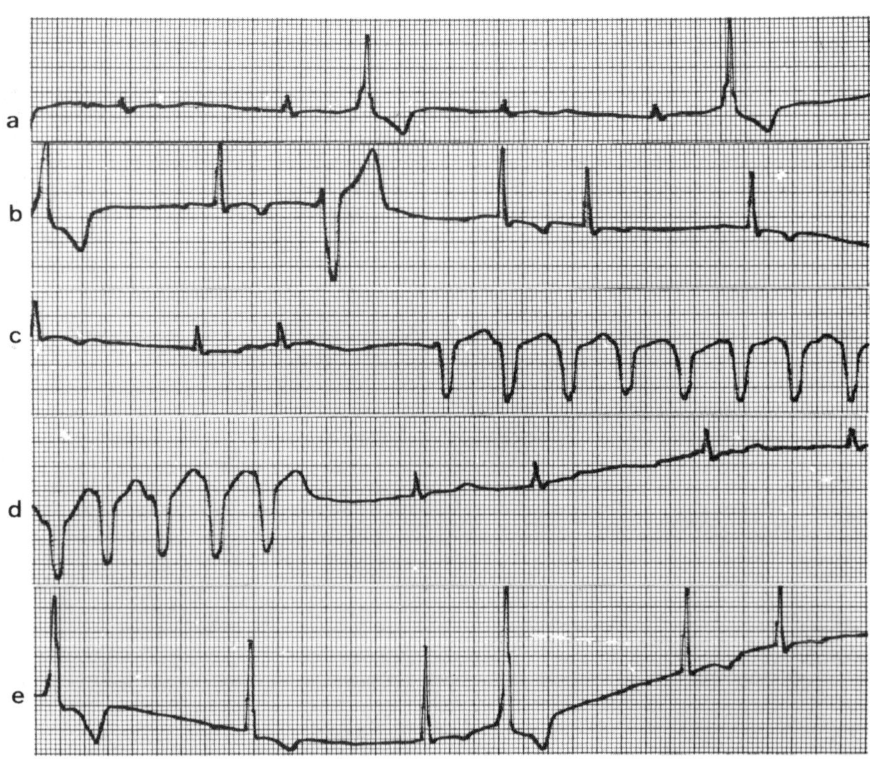

FIGURE 4-2. These Holter monitor ECG rhythm strips **a** to **e** are not continuous. The rhythm is sinus bradycardia with first degree A-V block, frequent multifocal VPCs, and paroxysmal VT. These ECG findings represent bradytachyarrhythmia syndrome as a manifestation of advanced SSS.

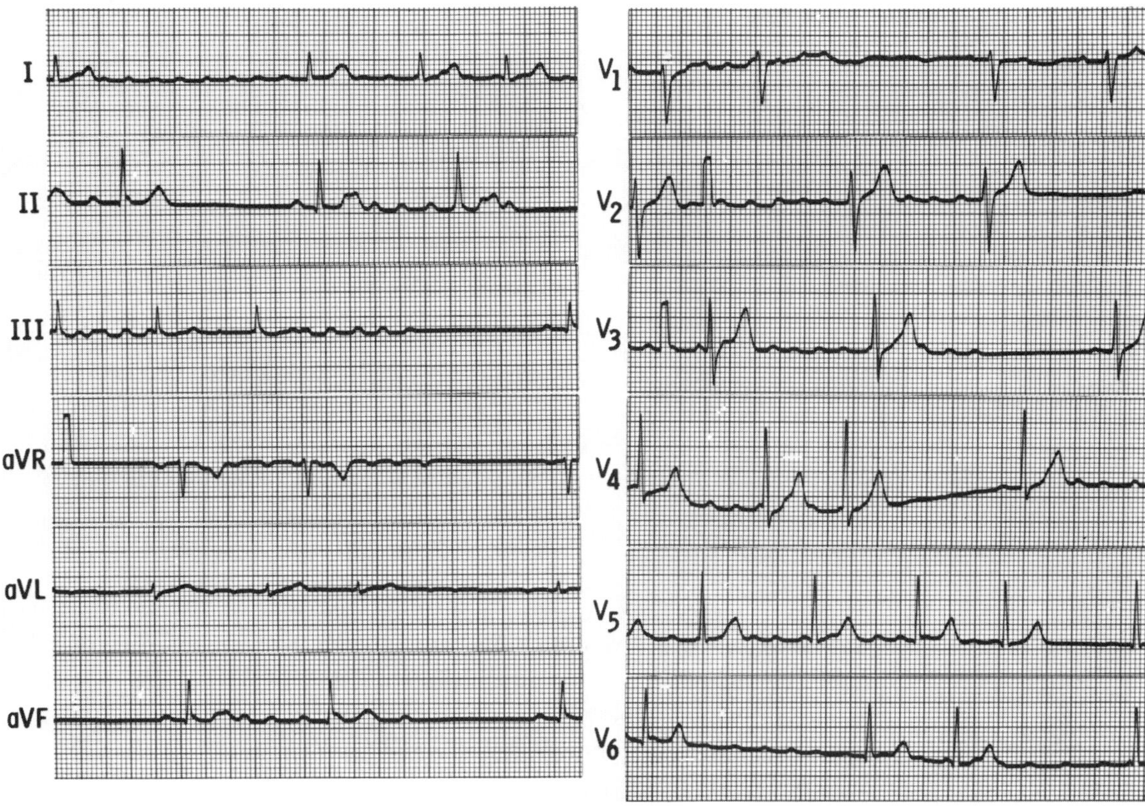

FIGURE 4-3. SSS is manifested by sinus bradycardia and intermittent atrial flutter with advanced A-V block leading to a very slow ventricular rate.

cycle. On the other hand, Mobitz type I (Wenckebach) S-A block produces a progressive shortening of the P-P cycles until a pause occurs. Mobitz type I (Wenckebach) S-A block is analogous to the Mobitz type I (Wenckebach) A-V block, whereas Mobitz type II S-A block is analogous to the Mobitz type II A-V block.

5. In cases of far-advanced S-A block or sinus arrest, the sinus activity is almost completely, or at times entirely, absent—leading to atrial standstill.

6. When the basic sinus cycle is irregular, it is impossible to distinguish between sinus arrest and S-A block.

Drug-Resistant Sinus Bradyarrhythmias

1. When a sinus bradyarrhythmia fails to respond to atropine or isoproterenol (Isuprel), the diagnosis of SSS is almost certain.

2. The diagnosis of SSS is usually entertained if the sinus rate is not accelerated beyond 90 beats/min after intravenous injection of atropine sulfate (1 to 2 mg).

3. For a similar reason, SSS can be diagnosed when intravenous

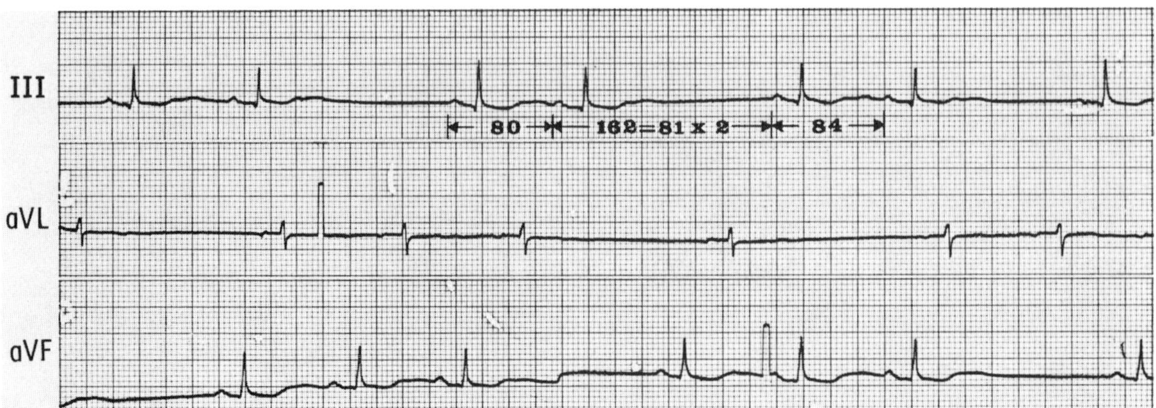

FIGURE 4-4. Sinus rhythm with intermittent Mobitz type II S-A block. (The numbers represent hundredths of a second.) This ECG finding is a manifestation of SSS.

isoproterenol (1 to 2 mg/min) fails to enhance the sinus rate beyond 90 to 100 beats/min in sinus bradycardia.

4. It should be noted that isoproterenol administration may provoke ventricular tachyarrhythmias.

Long Pause After an Atrial Premature Contraction

In general, an atrial premature contraction is *not* followed by a full compensatory pause because the sinus node is passively activated by the ectopic atrial impulse. Thus the automaticity of the sinus node is momentarily disturbed by the ectopic atrial impulse. Occasionally, an APC is followed by a full compensatory pause when the APC occurs during the late cardiac cycle so that the sinus node impulse formation is not disturbed. In this case, the interference (collision) between the sinus impulse and the ectopic atrial impulse occurs at the S-A junction, in the atria, or at the A-V junction. Extremely rarely, an APC is interpolated.

1. Although a postectopic pause after an APC is *not* fully compensatory, the returning cycle (the interval from the ectopic P wave to the first sinus P wave) is usually longer than the basic sinus P-P cycle because of transient suppression of the sinus node by the ectopic atrial impulse—a physiological phenomenon.

2. When the returning cycle is longer than usual, however, an abnormally prolonged refractory period of the sinus node is suspected.

3. In cases of a markedly prolonged sinus node recovery time caused by SSS, a single APC may be sufficient to produce sinus arrest, leading to the absence of the sinus P waves for a long period of time (Figure 4-5).

4. The A-V junctional or ventricular escape rhythm frequently seems to activate the ventricles under this circumstance (Figure 4-5).

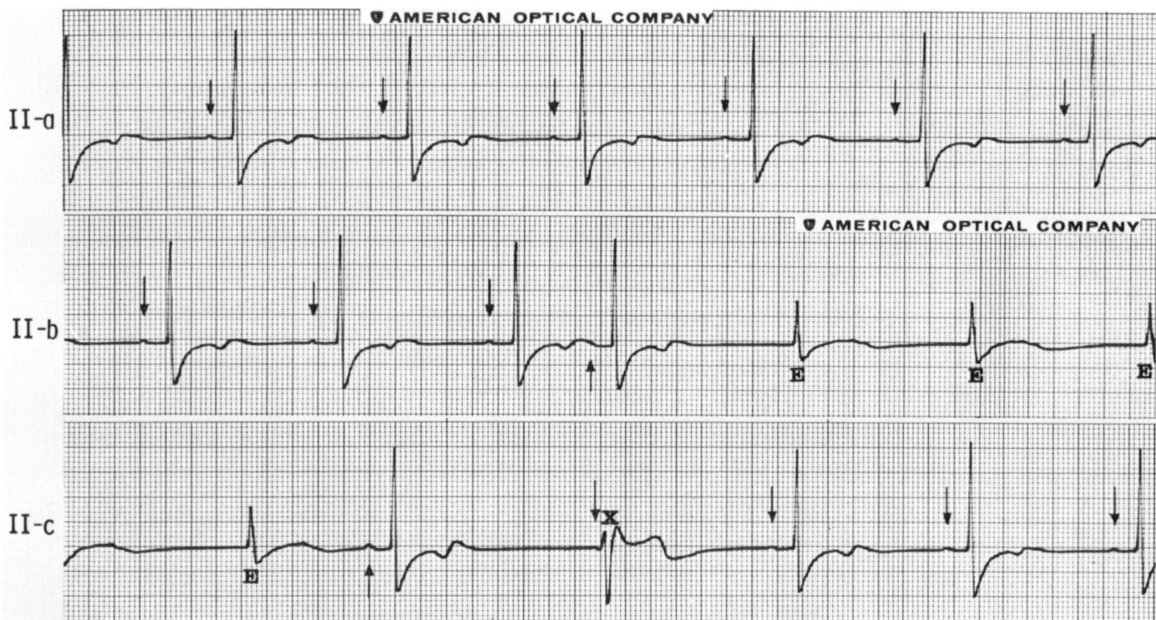

FIGURE 4-5. Sinus bradycardia (*downward arrows*) with occasional APCs (*upward arrows*) leading to ventricular escape rhythm (*E*) as a result of sinus arrest. Note the ventricular escape beat arising from another focus (*X*). These ECG findings represent advanced SSS. Leads II-a, II-b, and II-c are continuous.

Prolonged Sinus Node Recovery Time Determined by Atrial Pacing

The prolonged sinus node recovery time determined by rapid atrial pacing (rate: 120 to 150 beats/min) is a reliable indicator for the SSS. Rapid atrial pacing is particularly valuable when the ECG manifestations of SSS are not obvious and the clinical symptoms are vague. Detailed descriptions regarding determination of the sinus node recovery time and its usefulness are found later in this chapter (see Diagnostic Approach).

Chronic or Repetitive AF (Less Commonly, Atrial Flutter)

1. Chronic AF is the most common underlying rhythm in patients with far-advanced SSS; if this is the case, the sinus node is no longer capable of producing the cardiac impulse.

2. In such cases, AF is often associated with a slow ventricular rate (rate: 30 to 50 beats/min) as a result of advanced A-V block, and one or more A-V junctional (less commonly ventricular) escape beats may occur.

3. Until AF is well established as a chronic form, it is often preceded or followed by marked sinus bradycardia, sinus arrest, or S-A block, with or without first degree A-V block (see Figure 1-6).

4. Less commonly, atrial flutter is the underlying rhythm in ad-

vanced SSS, and again the ventricular rate is often slow because of advanced A-V block (Figure 4-6).

5. Until atrial flutter is well established, it is often preceded or followed by marked sinus bradycardia, sinus arrest, or S-A block in SSS.

6. In some cases of SSS, however, the ventricular rate is relatively fast in atrial fibrillation or flutter, leading to BTS (see Figure 1-6).

A-V Junctional Escape Rhythm (With or Without Slow and Unstable Sinus Activity)

1. When marked sinus bradycardia is further deteriorated, it is often followed by sinus arrest, and A-V junctional escape rhythm may become the underlying rhythm with or without any unstable sinus activity (Figure 4-7).

2. A-V junctional escape rhythm is commonly irregular until it becomes well established in its chronic form.

3. In chronic A-V junctional escape rhythm the cycle is usually regular.

4. Under this circumstancc, rctrogradc P waves may be preceded or followed by QRS complexes, and at times no P wave is discernible (Figure 4-7).

Carotid Sinus Syncope

It has been reported that sudden development of sinus arrest by carotid sinus stimulation lasting more than 3 sec is highly suggestive of inappropriate sinus node responsiveness—SSS (Figure 4-8). Similarly, the

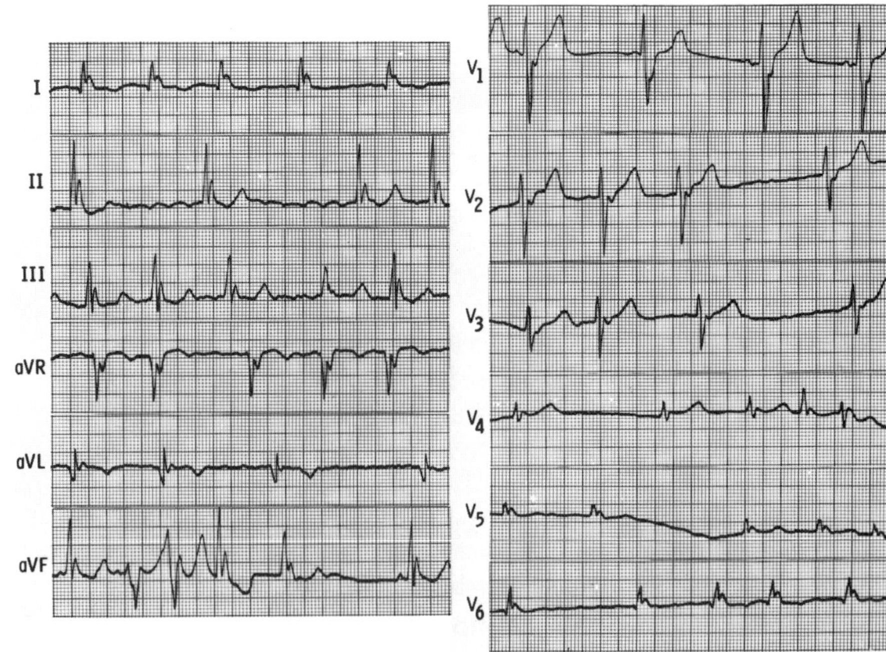

FIGURE 4-6. SSS is manifested by a very unstable sinus bradycardia (lead V_1) and intermittent atrial flutter-fibrillation with advanced A-V block causing a slow ventricular rate. Note the evidence of posterolateral MI associated with diffuse (nonspecific) intraventricular block. There are also frequent VPCs with group beats (lead aVF).

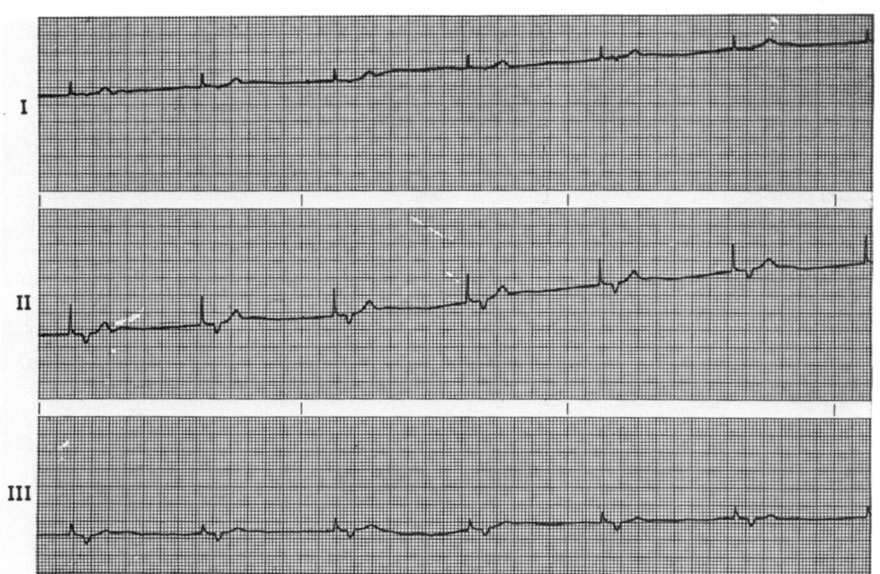

FIGURE 4-7. SSS is manifested by an A-V junctional escape rhythm. Note that each QRS complex is followed by a retrograde P wave.

appearance of long ventricular standstill in chronic atrial fibrillation or flutter induced by carotid sinus stimulation probably has the same clinical significance.

Failure of Restoration of Sinus Rhythm After Cardioversion

SSS is strongly suspected when there is an inability of the heart to restore a stable sinus rhythm for a long period of time after the termination of any ectopic tachyarrhythmia by direct current (DC) shock. This is particularly true after the termination of atrial fibrillation or flutter. Under this circumstance, A-V junctional escape rhythm becomes the dominant

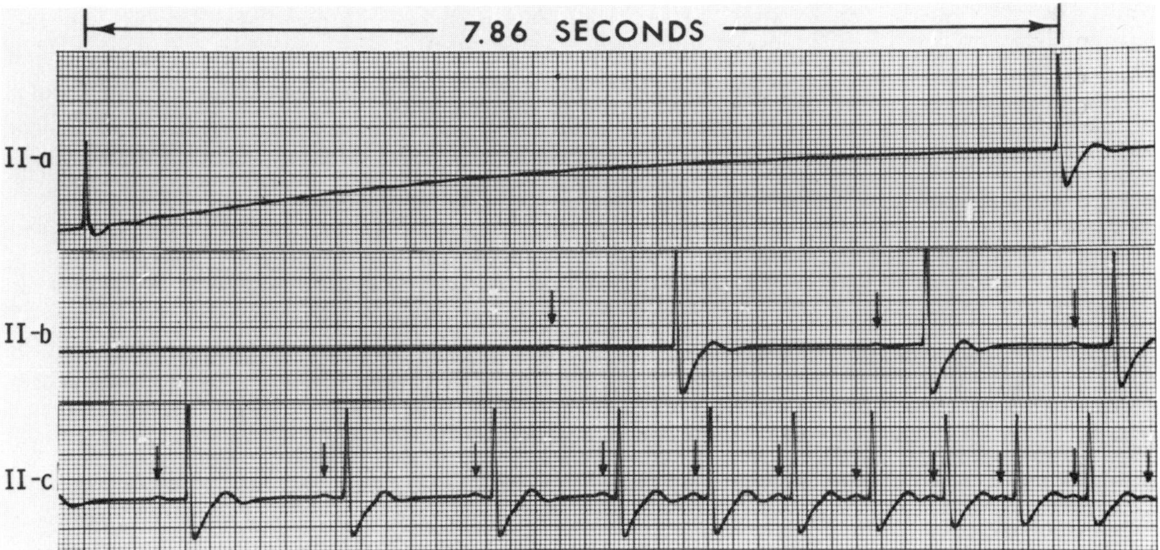

FIGURE 4-8. Leads II-a, II-b, II-c are continuous. *Arrows* indicate sinus P waves. Carotid sinus syncope is manifested by sinus arrest (7.86 sec) with occasional A-V junctional escape beats.

rhythm in many cases with or without unstable sinus P waves. In far-advanced SSS, AF may persist with unstable A-V junctional or ventricular escape rhythm after the termination of ventricular tachyarrhythmias by DC shock.

Bradytachyarrhythmia Syndrome

Although some investigators use the terms bradytachyarrhythmia syndrome and SSS interchangeably, these conditions are by no means identical. It must be reemphasized that the BTS is one of the common manifestations of advanced SSS.

1. In BTS the bradyarrhythmia component is commonly marked sinus bradycardia and less commonly chronic AF with a slow ventricular rate.
2. The most common tachyarrhythmia component in BTS is AF with a rapid ventricular response (see Figure 1-6) and less commonly atrial flutter with a rapid (often 2:1) ventricular response.
3. Paroxysmal atrial tachycardia (PAT) or A-V junctional tachycardia as a tachyarrhythmia component in BTS is not common.
4. The incidence of ventricular tachyarrhythmia in BTS has been reported to be 8 to 10% by different authors (see Figure 4-2).

Common Coexisting A-V Block and/or Intraventricular Block

Although A-V block or intraventricular block per se is *not* a part of SSS, these conditions often coexist because of the same underlying disease process; degenerative-sclerotic change may involve diffusely the entire conduction system. This is the reason advanced or even complete A-V block often occurs in patients with chronic atrial fibrillation or flutter, leading to a very slow ventricular rate in advanced SSS. In addition, first degree A-V block (P-R interval greater than 0.24 sec) is extremely common in BTS, and it is often preceded or followed by AF with a slow ventricular rate. Furthermore, various forms of intraventricular block frequently coexist with SSS (Figure 4-6).

Any Combination of the Above Findings

As can be expected, various ECG manifestations of SSS itself may be present, or common coexisting ECG abnormalities (e.g., A-V block, intraventricular block, A-V junctional or ventricular escape rhythm) may occur together with the SSS. For example, one ECG tracing with advanced SSS may consist of marked sinus bradycardia, sinus arrest, A-V junctional as well as ventricular escape beats, paroxysmal AF, and ventricular premature contractions (see Figure 1-6). Another form of SSS may be manifested by sinus bradycardia, intermittent S-A block, left bundle branch block, and ventricular escape beats.

CLINICAL CONSIDERATIONS

Laslett offered the original report concerning syncopal attacks associated with bradycardia in 1909. Interest and awareness of the therapeutic problems regarding SSS and BTS have increased among physicians since Short described the therapeutic dilemma in patients presenting with sinus bradycardia and tachyarrhythmia associated with syncope.

The clinical manifestations in patients with SSS are fundamentally caused by hypoperfusion of the vital organs, particularly the brain, heart, and kidney as a result of a markedly slow ventricular rate which may or may not be associated with tachyarrhythmias.

Sex and Age

There is no particular sexual preponderance for SSS, but the syndrome has been reported among elderly females more frequently than among elderly males.

1. SSS may involve any age group, although the syndrome is primarily a disease of elderly individuals.
2. The peak incidence of SSS has been reported to be during the sixth and seventh decades of life.
3. It has been suggested that SSS may be the cause of sudden death in some young athletes.
4. Another recent report described eight Africans with SSS, all of whom were age 32 or younger.
5. Recent literature indicates that SSS is not uncommon among young people in some parts of the world. The life expectancy in different parts of the world seems to influence greatly the peak incidence of SSS.

Underlying Heart Disease

1. The most common underlying heart disease in SSS has been reported to be CAD (about 50% incidence).
2. The next most common underlying disease process seems to be idiopathic: sclerotic-degenerative change in the sinus node and other conduction system (an incidence of about 30 to 35%).
3. Of course, many patients with SSS may have more than one underlying cardiac disease.
4. Less common underlying diseases of SSS include RHD, congenital heart disease, hypertension, cardiomyopathy, amyloidosis, hemochromatosis, surgical injury, myocarditis, pericarditis, Friedreich's ataxia, progressive muscular dystrophy, collagen disease, and metastatic disease.

Clinical Manifestations

Clinical manifestations of SSS may be multifaceted, and they may occur only intermittently. The most common manifestations of advanced SSS are lightheadedness and near or actual syncope; however, in mild cases the patient may be totally asymptomatic. In its early stage, the disease may be extremely difficult to recognize or evaluate.

Cerebral Manifestations

1. In mild cases or in the early stage of SSS, diminished cerebral arterial blood flow may manifest by generalized fatigue, muscle ache, or slight personality changes, including irritability, intermittent memory loss, and insomnia.

2. When SSS is further developed, cerebral manifestations may include slurred speech, pareses, erroneous judgment, lightheadedness, and near-syncope followed by actual fainting episodes.

3. Severe cerebral manifestations, e.g., syncope or near-syncope, are almost always caused by marked slowing of the heart rate or cardiac arrest, and the tachycardia component seldom produces significant cerebral symptoms.

4. Because the SSS is primarily a disease of elderly individuals, the various cerebral manifestations are frequently misinterpreted as cerebrovascular accidents or simply as senility.

5. Syncope or near-syncope has been reported to occur in 40 to 70% of patients with SSS; the incidence of dizziness is reported to be 6 to 7%.

Cardiac Manifestations

Various cardiac manifestations are the second most common finding in SSS.

1. In the early stage of mild SSS, cardiac manifestations other than a slow heart rate or a mixture of slow and rapid cardiac rhythms may be completely absent.

2. The three most common cardiac manifestations in SSS include palpitations, increased signs of CHF, and increased angina.

3. In some instances a sudden occurrence of, or episodic, acute pulmonary edema may be the first sign of SSS because the patient may not seek the medical attention during the mild stage of the syndrome.

4. Palpitations may be caused by an extremely slow rhythm (e.g., sinus bradycardia or AF with advanced A-V block), an irregular rhythm, or a mixture of slow and rapid rhythms (BTS).

5. Most patients experience palpitations when the cardiac rhythm suddenly changes—from a slow rhythm to a rapid rhythm or vice versa.

6. The three common cardiac manifestations (palpitations, angina, and CHF) of SSS are interrelated, and one symptom frequently aggravates the others.

7. In far-advanced cases of SSS, the patients may develop prolonged cardiac arrest or ventricular fibrillation leading to death.

Other Manifestations

Various nonspecific manifestations, e.g., oliguria or gastrointestinal distress) are not uncommon in SSS, but these findings are usually secondary to hypoperfusion to the heart itself.

DIAGNOSTIC APPROACH

It is not always easy to diagnose mild cases of SSS with any certainty. A high index of suspicion is often necessary to reach the correct diagnosis during the early stage of the disease. Marked and persisting sinus bradycardia (*not* caused by drugs) should always raise the possibility of SSS even in totally asymptomatic young individuals, including athletes.

Clinical Manifestations

The diagnosis of SSS (Table 4-2) cannot be made with any certainty by recognizing clinical findings alone. However, the disorder must be included in the differential diagnosis when the patient has a history of syncope or near-syncope. Similarly, SSS should be suspected as a possible underlying disorder in any individual with unexplainable pulmonary edema, palpitations, or angina, particularly when these findings (singly or together) are associated with a slow heart rate not caused by drugs (e.g., digitalis, propranolol).

Routine 12-Lead ECG

The diagnosis of advanced SSS can be confirmed by typical ECG findings shown on a routine 12-lead ECG or long rhythm strips.

Ambulatory (Holter Monitor) ECG

When the typical ECG findings of SSS are not documented on the routine 12-lead ECG because the finding is intermittent, the Holter monitor ECG is the best diagnostic tool.

Carotid Sinus Stimulation and Valsalva Maneuver

Sinus arrest lasting more than 3 sec with carotid sinus stimulation is strongly suggestive of inappropriate sinus node responsiveness—SSS. As with carotid sinus stimulation, the patient's response to the Valsalva maneuver may be useful for demonstrating sinus node dysfunction: The

TABLE 4-2. Sick Sinus Syndrome: Diagnostic Approach

1. Clinical manifestations
2. Routine 12-lead ECG
3. Ambulatory (Holter monitor) ECG
4. Carotid sinus stimulation and Valsalva maneuver
5. Cardioversion
6. Exercise (stress) ECG test
7. Drugs (e.g., atropine, isoproterenol)
8. Electrophysiological studies
   a. Determination of sinus node recovery time by atrial pacing
   b. Determination of sinoatrial conduction time by atrial extrastimulus technique
   c. His bundle ECG

Valsalva maneuver produces the expected changes in aortic pulse pressure but causes little or no change in pulse rate. In contrast, the physiological bradycardia of the elderly demonstrates the expected acceleration of the heart rate during the strain phase (phase II) and the subsequent slowing of the heart rate during the blood pressure (BP) overshoot (phase IV). However, it should be noted that these procedures provide no direct diagnostic evidence of sinus node disease but give a clue to the functional status of the sinus node. Further investigation is often indicated.

Cardioversion

Needless to say, cardioversion is not a diagnostic method for SSS. However, failure of the sinus rhythm to be restored after termination of any ectopic tachyarrhythmia by the procedure is strongly diagnostic of SSS.

Exercise ECG Test

When the sinus rate does not increase significantly by the standard exercise ECG (e.g., treadmill) protocol, SSS may be suspected—providing that inappropriate sinus rate change is *not* influenced by drugs (e.g., propranolol). Of course, healthy individuals in good physical condition (e.g., daily runners, athletes) may not show a significant increment of the heart rate by the exercise ECG protocol simply because of insufficient workload rather than sinus node dysfunction.

Drugs

1. SSS is often suspected when the individual, particularly an elderly person, develops marked sinus bradycardia after administration of a small amount of digitalis or propranolol (Inderal); i.e., SSS may be unmasked by these drugs. However, the above finding is not sufficiently reliable for basing the diagnosis of SSS on it.

2. Recently, atropine has been used to evaluate the response of the sinus node. Physiological sinus bradycardia responds to the intravenous administration of atropine by a normal or exaggerated acceleration of the sinus rate.

3. In contrast, patients with SSS show no significant increment of the sinus rate after atropine administration.

4. It has been suggested that the diagnosis of SSS can be made when intravenous atropine sulfate (1 to 2 mg) fails to increase the sinus rate beyond 90 beats/min in sinus bradycardia and when the sinus node recovery time remains prolonged by rapid atrial pacing (pacing rate: 120 to 140 beats/min for 2 to 4 min after atropine injection.

5. Similarly, the diagnosis of SSS may be entertained when the sinus rate does not increase beyond 90 to 100 beats/min in sinus bradycardia after intravenous administration of isoproterenol (1 to 2 mg/min).

Electrophysiological Studies

Sinus Node Recovery Time

1. Among various electrophysiological studies, determination of the sinus node recovery time (postpacing pause) by rapid atrial pacing is the most reliable provocative test for obtaining indirect evidence of SSS.

2. It can be obtained by the use of a pervenous right atrial pacing catheter and conventional ECG recordings.

3. Artificial pacing can be performed by placing the catheter either within the coronary sinus or at the junction of the superior vena cava and right atrium, whichever location provides the most effective and consecutive atrial capture.

4. The initial pacing rate is usually 90 beats/min, and it is progressively increased thereafter by 10 beats/min every 2 to 4 min up to 150 beats/min.

5. The pacing is terminated suddenly at the end of each period, and the postpacing pause (the interval from the last pacing spike to the onset of the next sinus P wave) is measured.

6. When there is complete absence of the sinus P wave (atrial standstill) after the termination of pacing, the first A-V junctional escape interval is measured.

7. Atrial pacing must be restarted immediately, however, when there is complete cardiac arrest for 4 sec in order to avoid a syncopal episode.

8. The postpacing pause is expected to occur in individuals with a normal as well as a diseased sinus node, and this electrophysiological phenomenon is comparable to the posttachyarrhythmia pause. However, the diseased sinus node, needless to say, requires an abnormally long recovery time until the automaticity as a primary pacemaker is reestablished. Thus it has been documented that there is a clear distinction between normal and abnormal responses.

9. It has been reported that the actual sinus node recovery time after the termination of atrial pacing is closely related to the resting sinus rate—the slower the resting sinus rates, the longer the maximum postpacing pause.

10. When the resting sinus rate is between 75 and 85 beats/min, the maximum postpacing pause is estimated to be 115 and 128% of the resting cycle length (postpacing pause: 800 to 900 msec).

11. In sinus bradycardia (rate: 45 to 60 beats/min), the maximum postpacing pause is expected to be much longer, and abnormally prolonged sinus node suppression can be easily recognized.

12. In sinus rhythm with a rate of 60 beats/min (cycle length: 1,000 msec) the postpacing pause showing 125% of the resting value (1,250 msec) is strongly suggestive of SSS. The diagnosis of SSS is almost certain when the postpacing pause is longer than 1,250 msec in this circumstance.

13. When the resting sinus rate is 45 beats/min (cycle length: 1,420 msec), the postpacing pause of 1,700 msec or greater is diagnostic of

SSS, even though the percentage increase is only 120%. In severe SSS the postpacing pause may reach 2,000 to 6,000 msec.

Corrected Sinus Node Recovery Time
Narula et al. proposed the corrected sinus node recovery time (CSRT)—the difference between the postpacing pause and the resting sinus P-P cycle. The normal maximum CSRT is calculated to be 525 msec or less, whereas an abnormal CSRT is calculated to be 1,880 ± 1,079 msec.

Sinoatrial Conduction Time
By other methods of electrophysiological study, the sinoatrial conduction times (SACTs) were measured indirectly by atrial extrastimulus technique. In one study, prolonged (more than 152 msec) SACTs were associated with a high incidence of sinus node and/or atrial disease. On the other hand, others have reported that the SACT is not significantly different between control groups and patients with SSS.

His Bundle ECG
Because SSS is often associated with abnormalities in impulse formation and conduction elsewhere in the heart, the His bundle ECG can provide useful information. For example, abnormal electrophysiological properties within the A-V junction may indirectly support the diagnosis of SSS. In addition, by recognizing the coexisting conduction disturbance, a specific type of artificial pacing may be selected for a given patient with SSS.

THERAPEUTIC APPROACH

Antiarrhythmic drug therapy alone has been unsatisfactory in the treatment of SSS, and at present the use of a permanent artificial pacemaker is the treatment of choice for all patients with SSS. Drug therapy alone for SSS is unsuccessful for the following reasons:

1. The agent used for treating the tachyarrhythmia component is harmful for or aggravates the bradyarrhythmia component and vice versa.
2. There is a lack of therapeutic effects of pharmacological agents (e.g., atropine sulfate or isoproterenol) for bradyarrhythmias.
3. Many patients experience significant and intolerable side effects to the pharmacological agents.

It is generally agreed, therefore, that artificial pacemaker therapy is mandatory in almost every case of advanced SSS even if the patient is asymptomatic. In fact, at the present time the most common indication for an artificial pacemaker is SSS.

Artificial Pacemaker Therapy

1. The most ideal pacing mode for the majority of patients with SSS is bifocal (A-V sequential) demand pacing because many patients have coexisting A-V block.

2. In addition, the multiprogrammable pacemaker, which is a new artificial pacing design, is the most suitable for most patients with SSS because various pacemaker parameters (functions), e.g., the pacing rate and energy output, can be easily adjusted at any time after pacemaker implantation so that the pacemaker functions best suited for a given patient's clinical circumstance can be provided.

3. On the other hand, the ordinary demand ventricular pacemaker is quite satisfactory for many elderly patients with SSS.

4. When the atria are paced, the chance of suppressing various atrial tachyarrhythmias is much greater than pacing the ventricles in patients with BTS.

5. However, one or more antiarrhythmic agents may be indicated when the tachyarrhythmia component persists even after artificial pacing in BTS. Detailed descriptions regarding permanent artificial pacing are given in Chapter 8.

Antiarrhythmic Drug Therapy

1. As indicated earlier in the chapter, antiarrhythmic drug therapy alone is unsatisfactory and often hazardous for the patient with SSS. However, antiarrhythmic drug therapy can be instituted with relative safety after implantation of a permanent pacemaker.

2. Antiarrhythmic agents are often required for the patient with SSS because the tachyarrhythmia component is usually not suppressed by the pacing alone, although atrial pacing may be capable of eliminating atrial tachyarrhythmias.

3. Indications for specific antiarrhythmic agents are similar to those for the agents' use in various tachyarrhythmias which are not associated with SSS.

4. Digitalis is the drug of choice for atrial fibrillation or flutter or tachycardia with rapid ventricular response.

5. Digitalis and diurectics may improve myocardial function and indirectly suppress the atrial tachyarrhythmias in patients with the SSS associated with CHF.

6. At times, propranolol (Inderal) may be added when atrial tachyarrhythmias with rapid ventricular response are not well controlled by digitalis alone.

7. Quinidine is very useful for the prevention of atrial tachyarrhythmias.

8. When ventricular tachyarrhythmia is not controlled by artificial pacing, various drugs—e.g., procainamide (Pronestyl), quinidine, phenytoin (Dilantin), disopyramide phosphate (Norpace), or propranolol (Inderal)—may be tried as a single agent or as combination therapy.

9. Every physician should be clearly aware of the fact that no patient is immune to drug toxicity, particularly digitalis intoxication, even after artificial pacing (see Chapter 10).

PROGNOSIS

1. The natural course of diseases of the sinus node seems to be chronic, progressive, and long-standing, but it is difficult to determine the long-term prognosis with any certainty.

2. To our present knowledge, the diseased sinus node cannot be cured, and in most cases only symptomatic treatment with hemodynamic improvement—artificial pacing to replace the natural pacemaker—can provide a productive life for the patient with SSS.

3. The exact duration from the onset of the first manifestation of SSS until death is not known, but it seems to take many months to 5 to 10 years in most cases.

4. It will now be even more difficult to evaluate the natural course of SSS because of the ready availability of artificial pacemakers which are implanted in the early stage of the disease.

5. The danger of sudden death is always possible in untreated patients with SSS.

6. The initial stage of SSS is marked and chronic sinus bradycardia, which is followed progressively by the development of sinus arrest and/or sinoatrial block.

7. Advanced SSS is manifested by chronic atrial fibrillation or flutter with a slow ventricular rate caused by advanced A-V block and/or BTS.

8. Although chronic AF is considered to be the end stage of SSS, it is difficult to predict its appearance in every individual.

9. It is also difficult to predict the life expectancy of the individual with SSS after the development of chronic AF.

10. In a recent study dealing with 39 patients with SSS after pacemaker implantation, the long-term (6- to 59-month follow-up period) prognosis was reported to be poor; 15 patients (42%) died during the follow-up period in this study. Eleven of the 15 deaths (73%) were related to cardiac problems, but none was associated with either a cardiac arrhythmia or pacemaker failure. Symptoms recurred or persisted after pacemaker implantation in 14 patients, nine of whom died. Twenty-two patients became asymptomatic after pacing, and six of them died.

Temporary Pacing: Techniques

5

Temporary cardiac pacing was introduced as a lifesaving measure for the treatment of complete atrioventricular (A-V) block and other symptomatic bradyarrhythmias, e.g., sick sinus syndrome (SSS). Since then the indications for artificial pacing and the techniques available for its application have been greatly expanded. Temporary cardiac pacing requires access to the heart, a pulse generator capable of emitting a controlled electrical stimulus, and a conducting channel. Each of these aspects has been greatly developed since the advent of temporary pacing.

Pulse generators were originally relatively simple devices that discharged a small electrical current at an exact time interval. This proved unsatisfactory, however, and a second circuit system was added to provide feedback information from the cardiac cycle. Additional latitude has also been added in regard to the selection of rate and energy discharge.

Catheters have become more complex, particularly as diagnostic indications have been added, but they remain simple circuits through which electrical energy is both transmitted and sensed.

Temporary Cardiac Pacing

1. Temporary cardiac pacing may be undertaken for a variety of reasons, and the technique chosen may vary considerably with the purpose.

2. The indications for temporary pacing can be divided into urgent, semiurgent, and elective indications.

3. Those situations in which an abnormal cardiac rhythm results in hemodynamic compromise of vital organs (particularly the brain) constitute an urgent indication for artificial pacing. This usually occurs with the sudden onset of a severe bradyarrhythmia without the development of an adequate escape rhythm to maintain perfusion.

4. Acute myocardial infarction (MI) is a common clinical setting, but other situations include cardiomyopathies and intrinsic disease of the conduction system (e.g., SSS).

5. Less commonly, emergency cardiac pacing may be utilized as therapy for a life-threatening tachyarrhythmia. This may be accomplished by ''overdrive pacing'' or the use of antiarrhythmic drugs in conjunction with artificial pacing to prevent iatrogenic lethal bradyarrhythmias.

6. Regardless of the cardiac rhythm, if the hemodynamics are such that perfusion of vital organs is not critically compromised the situation is not urgent. This allows more time for pacemaker placement, and a safer method may be employed. Another benefit is that a more stable electrode position is often achieved. This situation occurs when a serious cardiac arrhythmia is threatened or present but severe hemodynamic compromise has not yet occurred.

7. The development of acute bifascicular (BFB) or trifascicular (TFB) block during acute MI, chronic complete A-V block, recurrent ectopic tachyarrhythmias, and advanced digitalis intoxication (DI) are some of the clinical situations in which semiurgent pacemaker placement may be considered.

8. Elective insertion of a temporary pacemaker occurs less commonly in most institutions than urgent or semiurgent insertion. Indications for elective placement include disorders such as SSS that are asymptomatic at the time of insertion in many cases.

9. Diagnostic atrial pacing as utilized for determining the angina threshold, His bundle electrocardiography, sinus node recovery time determinations, and programmed electrical stimulation for the evaluation of ventricular arrhythmias also fall into this category. In these situations the procedure can be planned far in advance.

Vascular Access Routes

1. Electrode contact with the myocardium may be accomplished through the venous or arterial systems or directly through the chest wall.

2. The venous system is the most commonly utilized route.

3. The arterial system should be avoided because of jeopardy to the circulation.

4. The transthoracic route is utilized only in extreme emergencies because it carries the greatest risk and is the least reliable. The one advantage of transthoracic pacing is that it can be accomplished very quickly.

5. The insertion of epicardial atrial and ventricular pacing wires during cardiac surgery may be considered a type of transthoracic temporary pacing. There is virtually no risk, however, and routine insertion after all open heart procedures should be encouraged. These wires are frequently helpful in postoperative management, and later placement under less favorable conditions may be avoided.

6. Four venous routes—brachial, jugular, subclavian, and femoral veins—have been routinely utilized. Each has advantages and disadvantages, the most important of which are summarized in Table 5-1.

TABLE 5-1. Sites of Entry for Temporary Artificial Pacing

Site	Percutaneous vs. Surgical Cutdown	Safety of Method	Patient Mobility
Brachial	Surgical cutdown	Very safe	Poor
Subclavian	Percutaneous	Potential hazard	Good
Jugular	Percutaneous or surgical cutdown	Safe	Good
Femoral	Percutaneous	Potential hazard	Very poor
Transthoracic	Percutaneous	Very hazardous (for emergency use only)	Not applicable

7. Hazards include the production of a pneumothorax or hemothorax with the subclavian approach, deep vein thrombosis with the femoral approach, and perforation of a coronary artery with the transthoracic approach.

8. The risks of any approach are less in experienced hands. The longer the catheter remains in place, the more important are patient mobility and catheter stability. Many physicians prefer the subclavian route because of these two considerations.

9. Less experienced operators encounter less risk using the brachial route. This approach, however, immobilizes the patient's arm and has a higher incidence of catheter dislocation.

10. The choice of entry site depends on the clinical circumstances, the anticipated length of time that artificial cardiac pacing will be needed, and the skill and experience of the operator.

Site Preparation and Entry

1. Good *skin preparation* and proper *sterile technique* are essential to minimize the chance of infection. The skin should be scrubbed twice over a wide area with an antiseptic solution, e.g., povidone-iodine or isopropyl alcohol. The entire operative field should then be draped with sterile towels or drapes to provide a large working area without risk of contamination to the instruments or the operator.

2. The technique of entry varies depending on whether the percutaneous approach or a venous cutdown is used.

3. In the *percutaneous method,* local anesthetic is infiltrated and a large-bore needle with a syringe attached is introduced into the vein.

4. One alternative is to use a needle with an external plastic catheter, advancing the catheter once there is blood return into the syringe, and then removing the needle. The pacing cathether can then be introduced though the plastic cathether.

5. The other alternative is to use a catheter sheath introducer system, which consists of a plastic catheter sheath with a valve on its proximal end and a side arm which is attached to an intravenous line to keep it flushed.

6. The valve prevents air from entering the catheter or fluid from leaking out and allows insertion and removal of the pacing catheter.

7. In the case of the jugular vein (which may also be approached via a cutdown), the skin is held taut by spreading it between the thumb and index finger. This helps to immobilize the vein and provides a fixed target.

8. The subclavian vein may be approached via the supra- or infraclavicular approach. The technique is illustrated in Figure 5-1A,B.

9. The femoral vein is located just medial to the femoral artery, which is located below the inguinal ligament.

10. The needle is inserted at an approximately 45-degree angle cephalad.

11. A small amount of aspiration can be applied to the syringe so that it yields blood as soon as the vein is entered.

12. Once the blood enters the syringe, the plastic cannula may be advanced while flow continues.

13. If no flow is seen, the needle is slowly withdrawn to determine if the vein has been punctured.

14. If it has not, the process is repeated.

15. The plastic cannula is then advanced carefully so that it remains within thc confines of the vein.

16. If a catheter sheath introducer system is used, the needle is introduced into the vein, the syringe is disconnected, a flexible guide wire is inserted through the needle, and the needle is removed.

17. The sheath and internal introducer are then passed into the vein over the guide wire.

18. The guide wire is then removed, the side arm is attached to an intravenous line, and the sheath is ready for insertion of the pacing catheter.

19. When a *venous cutdown* is utilized (brachial and occasionally jugular routes), a No. 15 scalpel blade is used to make a small (approximately 0.75 inch) incision over the vein.

20. The subcutaneous tissue is then spread with the use of straight and curved Kelly hemostats.

21. The vein is clearly exposed by blunt dissection and raised by placing a curved Kelly clamp beneath it.

22. Silk ties are placed under the vein at its most proximal and distal points of exposure.

23. The distal tie is tied, a small nick is made in the vein in the center of its exposed surface, and an introducer or eye forceps is placed in the lumen.

24. The pacing catheter is advanced below the instrument into the lumen of the vein.

25. With the *transthoracic emergency route* the skin is prepared and a puncture wound is made with a large-bore needle with an attached syringe.

26. The needle can be inserted into the fourth left intercostal space just lateral to the sternum, or it can be inserted from a subxiphoid position.

27. The syringe is disconnected, and a flexible pacing wire with a hooked end is inserted through the needle and then pulled back until it makes contact with the endocardial surface of the ventricle.

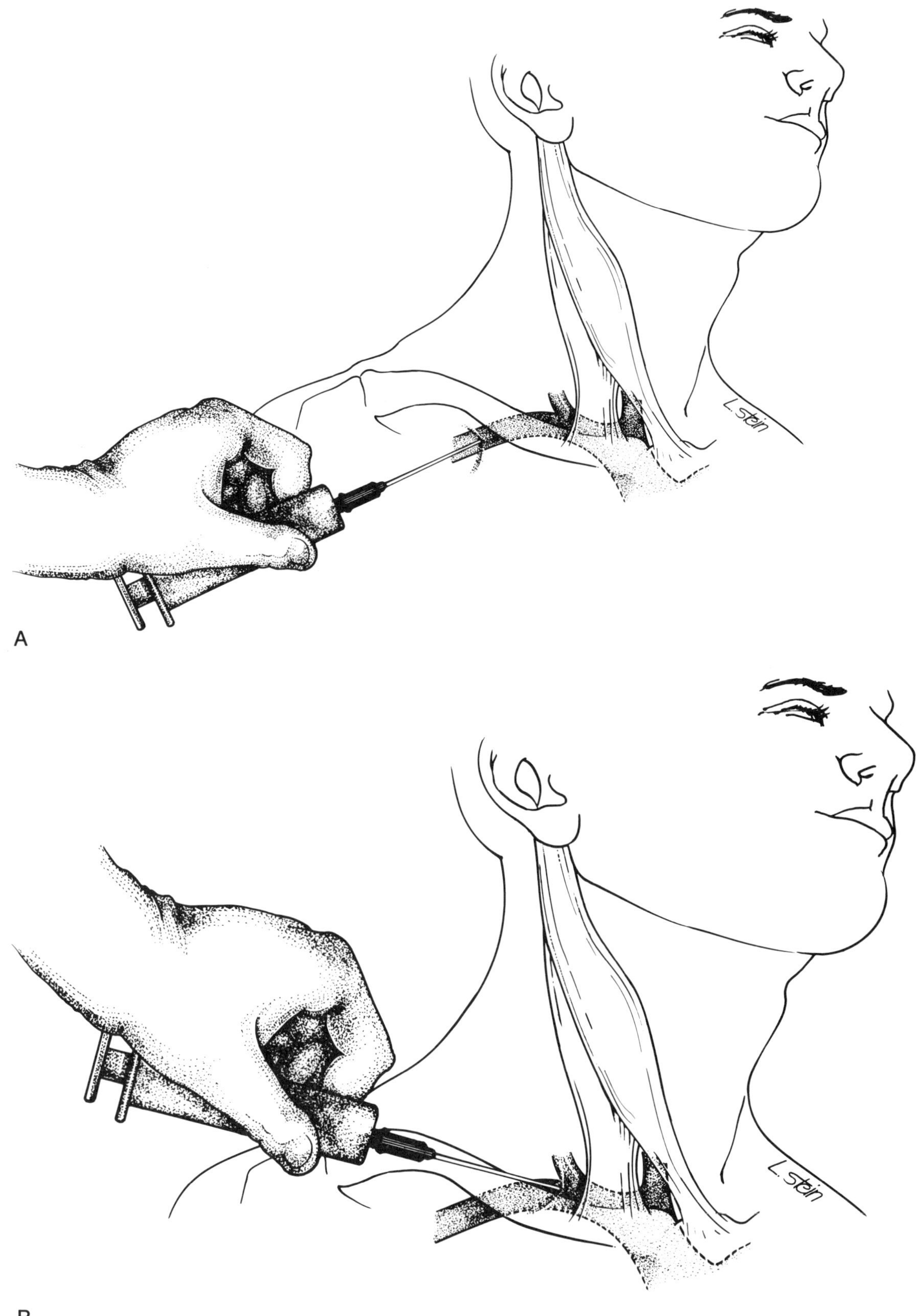

FIGURE 5-1. Cutaway illustrations demonstrate the infraclavicular **(A)** and supraclavicular **(B)** approaches to puncture of the subclavian vein in preparation for placement of a temporary pacemaker.

28. It should be stressed that this method is only for use in life-threatening situations where speed is critical.

29. The catheter should be replaced as soon as reasonably possible by a transvenous pacemaker.

Catheter Choice and Positioning

1. A wide variety of pacemaker cathethers are available that can be obtained in various sizes, usually ranging from 5 Fr to 7 Fr and with varying degrees of firmness.

2. Some physicians prefer a soft balloon-tipped, flow-directed catheter for insertion through the jugular or subclavian veins and passage to the right ventricle without fluoroscopy.

3. A Swan-Ganz pulmonary artery cathether with atrial and ventricular pacing electrodes is also available.

4. Others prefer firmer catheters inserted via the brachial or femoral veins under fluoroscopic guidance.

5. All catheters contain electrodes; unipolar catheters contain one electrode and bipolar catheters contain two.

6. Different catheters have varying distances between the electrodes, but these variations make little practical difference.

7. Most catheters today are bipolar; they can easily be converted to unipolar function simply by connecting one of the electrodes to the negative terminal of the battery and completing the circuit with an indifferent skin lead attached to the positive pole.

8. Bipolar pacing is more commonly used, but the advantage of unipolar pacing is that better sensing function is achieved in the demand mode.

9. The disadvantages of unipolar pacing include the necessity for an indifferent skin lead, a large pacing artifact on the electrocardiogram (ECG) which may be sensed by a monitoring device as an R wave of the QRS complex, and the occasional production of skin twitching. Several of these disadvantages may be avoided by using a special type of unipolar catheter that has a distal and a proximal electrode.

10. Although most pacemaker catheters contain no lumen, cathethers with a lumen can be obtained for positioning in the coronary sinus, where they can be used to pace the atrium and simultaneously collect blood samples.

11. When advancing the soft semifloating cathethers at the bedside, the leads are connected to standard ECG equipment and are monitored as the catheter is advanced.

12. A large inverted P wave is noted in the superior vena cava and upper right atrium. This becomes biphasic in the center of the right atrium and upright in the inferior portion of that chamber. As the tricuspid valve is crossed, the P wave becomes very small or disappears and a giant QRS complex appears. The catheter should then be advanced approximately 3 cm and pacing attempted. If pacing is not successful, the cathether should be withdrawn a short distance and then readvanced.

13. Firmer catheters in the brachial or femoral veins must be advanced under fluoroscopic guidance. This has the disadvantage of the patient needing to be moved (unless a portable fluoroscope is available) but has the advantage that the position of the cathether is visualized prior to termination of the procedure, thus increasing the likelihood of stability.

14. The catheter is passed blindly from its insertion in the brachial vein to the level of the shoulder. When occasional resistance is encountered, the catheter is withdrawn, rotated, and advanced. Fluoroscopic guidance is maintained from the level of the shoulder. The angle formed where the subclavian vein joins the brachiocephalic vein and where the latter enters the superior vena cava is sometimes rather acute and difficult to traverse, and visualization is required.

15. When the catheter is in the right atrium, the catheter tip may be directed toward the cardiac apex and can usually be passed into the right ventricle without difficulty.

16. In the posteroanterior view it may be difficult to discern the catheter position in the coronary sinus from the right ventricle. The catheter tends to "ride up" superiorly more in the coronary sinus, and no ventricular premature contractions (VPCs) are noted, although atrial premature contractions (APCs) may occur. The coronary sinus more nearly resembles the catheter position in the right ventricular outflow tract. However, if difficulty is encountered, the patient may be turned to the left anterior oblique projection where the right ventricle can be seen anteriorly and the coronary sinus posteriorly.

17. Once in the right ventricle, the tip of the catheter can usually be advanced to the right ventricular apex and flexed with slight pressure to assume the characteristic shape. Some physicians prefer to achieve this position by looping the cathether in the right atrium and rotating it. As it "flips" across the tricuspid valve, it usually takes up a position in the right ventricular outflow tract. From there it can be withdrawn until the tip is at the apex. This method is slightly more risky because of potential cardiac arrhythmias in the right ventricle, and it requires more skill. The former method is preferred.

18. When the approach is from the femoral vein, fluoroscopy is begun in the midabdomen. The natural curve of the catheter favors passage through the tricuspid valve, and it can usually be easily manipulated to the right ventricular apex.

Pulse Generators

As with the pacing catheters, several manufacturers supply external pulse generators, although the fundamental mode of operation is similar. Detailed descriptions regarding various methods of pacing and different types of pulse generators are found in Chapter 1.

1. When the artificial pacemaker is first placed in position, the threshold for capture should be carefully measured.

2. Not more than 0.7 to 1.0 milliamperes (mA) should be required if the pacemaker electrode is in a good position.

3. The threshold always increases during the first week of operation.

4. The initial setting should be approximately double the threshold.

5. It should be kept in mind that drugs such as propranolol (Inderal) also increase the threshold (see Chapter 9).

6. The optimal rate setting varies depending on the indication for artificial pacing and the individual's cardiovascular status.

7. Ideally, when pacing for complete A-V block, a pacing rate is selected that yields the best cardiac output. This can be easily assessed if a monitoring catheter is present in the pulmonary artery but otherwise must be judged clinically.

8. If overdrive of a cardiac arrhythmia is the goal, the pacing rate must reflect this, regardless of the cardiac output unless dangerous hemodynamic consequences are precipitated.

9. On occasion, e.g., when attempting to slow the ventricular response in a patient with atrial flutter, it may be desirable to pace the atrium at 400 to 1,000 beats/min. The ideal pacing rate can be adjusted easily when programmable pacemakers are used (see Chapter 1).

Maintenance and Malfunction

1. Having properly positioned an artificial pacemaker, one should secure it if it is to remain in place for a long period of time.

2. If entry was subcutaneous, the catheter may be attached at the skin line by a suture placed through the skin and tied about the catheter.

3. Approximately three skin sutures are then placed. No further sutures will be required upon withdrawal.

4. The skin is carefully cleansed and bandaged. Bandages are changed every 24 to 48 hr, and some physicians apply an antibiotic ointment. It should be stressed that good sterile care of the entry site will help to avoid serious future difficulty.

5. In most situations the underlying spontaneous (natural) cardiac rhythm should be checked at least every 24 hr. The recommended method is to gradually reduce the rate of the pulse generator until the spontaneous rate and rhythm become evident.

6. Pacemaker malfunction can occur in four places: the pulse generator, the catheter, the catheter-heart interface, or the heart itself. Electromechanical dissociation is the only way in which the heart itself may be the problem. This situation exists when the pacing impulse is appropriately applied to the endocardial surface and a resulting spike artifact and QRS complex are recorded but no myocardial contraction occurs. This is usually the result of severe end-stage myocardial ischemia, cardiomyopathy, or myocardial rupture and is almost invariably fatal.

7. The remaining three areas of potential difficulty (pulse generator, cathether, and catheter-heart interface) may best be approached by the process of elimination.

8. If a spike artifact is present on the ECG and the milliamperage is high enough for capture, then the catheter-heart interface is at fault. This usually means malposition or perforation.

9. In the absence of a spike artifact, the pulse generator or the catheter must be defective. This is determined by ascertaining the soundness of all connections and then replacing the pulse generator. If these maneuvers fail to correct the problem, the catheter must be defective.

10. Sensing failure is probably the most common cause of temporary pacemaker malfunction. The sensing circuit of a pacemaker requires a signal of sufficient amplitude and appropriate wave form (to avoid sensing large T waves, for instance) to recycle the discharge from the pulse generator.

11. The sensing function is usually less stable and more liable to malfunction than the pacing circuit. Thus minor degrees of malposition or increases in threshold may have no effect on pacing but may cause a failure of sensing because the circuit does not "see" a large enough QRS complex.

12. A failure of sensing may also occur during acute MI or with cardiomyopathy when the voltage of the QRS complex is markedly diminished. Repositioning is sometimes helpful; but when the amplitude of the QRS complex is insufficient, conversion to a unipolar system will permit the circuit to "see" a larger QRS complex. Detailed descriptions regarding malfunctions are found in Chapter 11.

Complications

Although there are many potential complications of temporary pacing, few are serious; and with reasonable care, injury to individuals can be kept to a minimum. No single complication occurs in more than a few percent of the cases that are performed competently. Detailed descriptions regarding various complications are found in Chapter 11.

Discontinuation of Pacing

1. Temporary artificial pacing is discontinued when it is no longer necessary or when a permanent pulse generator has been implanted.

2. Prior to removal, the cardiac rhythm should be observed for a reasonable length of time, with the pacemaker either off or well below the spontaneous rate. This helps ensure that an adequate rate and rhythm are present and that reinsertion will not be necessary.

3. If a permanent artificial pacemaker is to be placed, the temporary catheter and pulse generator should remain in place for 12 to 24 hr after the implantation in order to ensure normal function of the new generator.

4. The temporary pacing catheter should then be removed under fluoroscopic guidance to avoid any motion or displacement of the permanent wire.

5. If bleeding occurs at the site of entry, local pressure with sterile gauze is usually sufficient for control.

Temporary Pacing: Indications

6

It is extremely important to determine the indications versus the nonindications or contraindications of temporary cardiac pacing. One must weigh seriously the definite beneficial effect of temporary pacing against the potential risks which may directly or indirectly be involved with the procedure. The higher incidence of potential risks is expected when dealing with patients with acute myocardial infarction (MI) or myocardial ischemia. That is, the threshold for the initiation of ventricular fibrillation (VF) is proved to be significantly low during an acute ischemic event leading to VF or even death during or immediately after temporary pacing (see Chapter 11).

When permanent cardiac pacing is considered to be indicated (see Chapter 8), it can be carried out directly as an elective surgery so long as the patient is asymptomatic, and potential danger from the arrhythmia itself is unlikely present without temporary pacing. On the other hand, temporary pacing is indicated when significant symptoms (e.g., near or actual syncope, hypotension) caused by the arrhythmia are present prior to permanent pacemaker implantation.

The precise criteria for the use of a temporary or a permanent cardiac pacemaker vary slightly from one institution to another and among physicians. The generally accepted criteria for temporary pacing are summarized in Table 6-1. As described elsewhere in this book, a major controversy exists among physicians regarding the use of prophylactic pacing in patients with acute MI (see Chapter 7).

There are three major factors which determine the indications of temporary pacing: (1) symptoms (e.g., dizziness, near-syncope, syncope, hypotension, heart failure); (2) ventricular rate; and (3) clinical circumstances (underlying heart disease or a direct cause of the arrhythmia). In general, a ventricular rate below 40 beats/min requires temporary pacing, and in most cases the patient is often symptomatic in this circumstance. In regard to the clinical circumstances, acute arrhythmia often requires

TABLE 6-1. Indications of Temporary Pacing

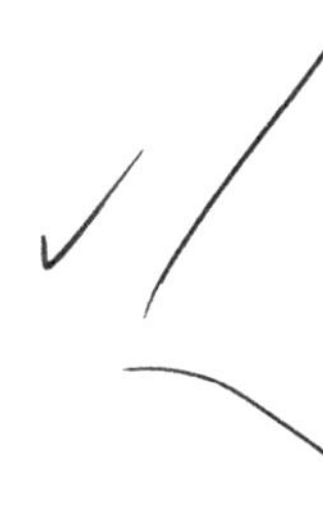

1. Symptomatic second degree, high degree, and complete A-V block
2. Symptomatic bradyarrhythmias due to any mechanism resulting from acute MI
3. Acute bifascicular or trifascicular block due to acute MI
4. Sick sinus syndrome and bradytachyarrhythmia syndrome
5. Symptomatic digitalis-induced bradyarrhythmias
6. Drug-resistant tachyarrhythmias
7. Carotid sinus syncope (often due to SSS)
8. Ventricular standstill
9. Before or during implantation of a permanent pacemaker
10. Prophylactic pacing during and immediately after major cardiac surgery when significant bradyarrhythmias are anticipated

temporary pacing more often than chronic arrhythmia. This is particularly true when dealing with acute arrhythmias associated with recent MI (see Chapter 7).

VARIOUS CLINICAL CIRCUMSTANCES

Symptomatic Second Degree, High Degree, and Complete A-V Block

1. Two major factors influence the indications versus nonindications of temporary pacing in second degree, high degree (advanced), and complete (third degree) atrioventricular (A-V) block. The first factor is the symptoms, which include dizziness, near-syncope, syncope, hypotension, and congestive heart failure. The second factor is the ventricular rate.

2. When the ventricular rate is 40 beats/min or less in 2:1 A-V block, the patient is nearly always symptomatic (see Figure 2-3) regardless of whether the block is in the A-V nodal (intranodal) or infranodal region.

3. A 2:1 A-V block caused by A-V nodal block is often found in patients with digitalis intoxication (DI) or acute diaphragmatic MI.

4. When 2:1 A-V block is found to be a variant of Mobitz type II A-V block (infranodal block; see Figure 2-3 and Chapter 2), a permanent pacemaker is indicated. It may be necessary to insert a temporary pacemaker before permanent pacemaker implantation in this circumstance when the patient is significantly symptomatic (e.g., has syncope or near-syncope).

5. In Wenckebach (Mobitz type I) A-V block, temporary pacing is unlikely to be indicated unless the patient is symptomatic or the ventricular rate is slower than 40 beats/min. Wenckebach A-V block is commonly caused by DI (see Chapter 2).

6. In high degree (advanced) or complete (third degree) A-V block, again the symptoms and ventricular rate are the determining factors.

7. Transient (reversible) advanced or complete A-V block is usually A-V nodal block which is commonly caused by acute diaphragmatic MI or DI.

8. Infranodal advanced or complete A-V block (trifascicular block)

always requires permanent pacing regardless of the clinical circumstances. Temporary pacing may be needed before implantation of a permanent pacemaker—depending on the ventricular rate and the presence or severity of symptoms, particularly near-syncope or syncope.

Symptomatic Bradyarrhythmias by any Mechanism Resulting from Acute MI

In most patients with acute diaphragmatic MI, bradyarrhythmias are usually transient and seldom require artificial pacing. On the other hand, artificial pacing is often required in patients with anterior MI because A-V block under this circumstance is usually irreversible. Prophylactic pacing is frequently used in those with anterior MI. Detailed descriptions regarding artificial pacing in MI are found in Chapter 7.

Acute Bifascicular or Trifascicular Block Caused by Acute MI

There is significant controversy among physicians regarding the use of artificial pacemakers in patients with acute MI. This is particularly true when dealing with prophylactic pacing in acute MI. It is generally agreed, however, that prophylactic temporary pacing is indicated for acute bifascicular block (BFB) or incomplete trifascicular block (TFB) caused by acute MI (see Figure 2-5). Detailed descriptions regarding prophylactic pacing in patients with acute MI are found in Chapter 7.

Sick Sinus Syndrome and Bradytachyarrhythmia Syndrome

Advanced sick sinus syndrome (SSS) (Figures 1-6, 4-2, 4-3, and 4-6) eventually requires permanent pacing because antiarrhythmic drug therapy alone is unsatisfactory. In some cases, one or more antiarrhythmic agents are necessary when the tachyarrhythmia component is not suppressed by the artificial pacing. Bradytachyarrhythmia syndrome is often a manifestation of advanced SSS (Figures 1-6, 4-2, and 4-3). However, some patients with bradytachyarrhythmia syndrome (see Figure 2-7) are *not* caused by SSS.

Temporary pacing is necessary before permanent pacemaker implantation when the patient is symptomatic (e.g., has near-syncope or syncope) with SSS. Detailed descriptions regarding SSS are found in Chapter 4.

Symptomatic Digitalis-Induced Bradyarrhythmias

As repeatedly emphasized, no one is immune to DI even after pacing (see Chapter 10). On the other hand, artificial pacing (usually temporary) may be indicated when the patient develops symptomatic and marked bradyarrhythmias caused by DI. Digitalis-induced bradyarrhythmias may be marked sinus bradycardia, sinus arrest, or sinoatrial (S-A) block, but they are commonly second degree, advanced, or complete A-V block. In many cases the atrial mechanism is atrial tachyarrhythmias including fibrillation, flutter, or tachycardia in these circumstances. As a rule, a permanent pacemaker is *not* indicated for digitalis-induced bradyarrhythmias.

Drug-Resistant Tachyarrhythmias

1. When ectopic tachyarrhythmias, particularly ventricular tachycardia (VT), become refractory to antiarrhythmic drug therapy and/or direct current shock, artificial pacing with an overdriving pacing rate (80 to 120 beats/min) is indicated.

2. Various modes of artificial pacing may be used for the treatment of refractory tachyarrhythmias (see Chapter 1), but atrial or coronary sinus pacing is often ideal for temporary pacing, particularly when the atrial contribution is essential to maintain adequate cardiac output (see Figure 1-7).

3. When there is significant coexisting A-V block, bifocal pacing should be carried out (see Figure 1-5).

Carotid Sinus Syncope

1. Artificial pacing is definitely indicated for any individual who develops marked slowing of the ventricular rate as a result of a hypersensitive reaction to carotid sinus stimulation.

2. Many patients with carotid sinus syncope develop near-syncope or syncope resulting from marked sinus bradycardia, advanced A-V block, or ventricular standstill (see Figure 4-8) by slight compression on the carotid sinus area (e.g., shaving, rotation of neck, tight collar, wearing a necktie). Under these circumstances, permanent pacing is indicated.

3. In some cases, however, hypersensitive reactions to carotid sinus stimulation may be markedly exaggerated by administration of digitalis, methyldopa (Aldomet), guanethidine (Ismelin), and propranolol (Inderal). Temporary pacing may be indicated in addition to the withdrawal of the causative agent when the carotid sinus syncope is considered to be primarily drug-induced.

4. Carotid sinus syncope is often a manifestation of SSS (see Figure 4-8), and permanent pacing is indicated under this circumstance (see Chapters 4 and 8).

Ventricular Standstill

1. Permanent pacing is usually indicated for spontaneous ventricular standstill.

2. Ventricular standstill, of course, may be an expression of a hypersensitive reaction to carotid sinus stimulation (see above), but it may also be totally unexplainable.

3. Ventricular standstill may be a manifestation of SSS (see Chapter 4).

4. Ventricular standstill may be drug-induced (e.g., digitalis toxicity), or it may be a result of electrolyte imbalance (e.g., hyperkalemia).

5. When the direct causative factor is found, it should be corrected immediately. In this case, temporary pacing may be required if the ventricular standstill is symptomatic.

Before or During Implantation of a Permanent Pacemaker

Permanent pacemaker implantation may be carried out directly as an elective procedure when the bradyarrhythmia is found to be chronic and when the patient is relatively asymptomatic. On the other hand, temporary pacing is essential before permanent pacemaker implantation when the arrhythmia develops acutely, especially during acute MI and/or when the arrhythmia produces significant symptoms (e.g., near-syncope or syncope).

Prophylactic Pacing During and Immediately After Major Cardiac Surgery

Temporary prophylactic pacing may be indicated during and immediately after major cardiac surgery when there is a potential danger of developing significant bradyarrhythmias. For example, prophylactic pacing will definitely be beneficial when: (1) the patient is elderly; (2) the cardiac rhythm tends to be unstable; (3) the preoperative electrocardiogram (ECG) shows BFB or incomplete TFB; or (4) the cardiac conduction tissue is likely to be damaged during surgery. Some cardiac surgeons prophylactically pace all patients routinely during major cardiac surgery, but this view is not uniformly accepted.

Artificial Pacing and Acute Myocardial Infarction

7

There is significant controversy among physicians regarding the use of artificial pacemakers for patients with acute myocardial infarction (MI), a controversy that involves the use of temporary as well as permanent pacing. Prophylactic pacing always creates profound controversy. The main reason for the controversy is that there are multiple factors which influence the morbidity and mortality of patients with acute MI. Thus the value of artificial pacing is often difficult to evaluate because many patients with acute MI die from complications—e.g., congestive heart failure (CHF) and cardiogenic shock—as well as from cardiac rhythm problems with or without artificial pacing. Moreover, it is frequently uncertain whether the conduction abnormalities, particularly bundle branch block (BBB) and bifascicular (BFB) or trifascicular (TFB) blocks, were present before acute MI or the MI actually produced these conduction disturbances. The morbidity and mortality seem to be much worse in patients in whom these fascicular blocks are produced acutely by recent MI in comparison to those patients who had the fascicular blocks before the acute MI.

In certain clinical situations, e.g., Mobitz type II atrioventricular (A-V) block or acute BFB or TFB in acute MI, it is generally agreed that artificial pacing is definitely indicated. Artificial pacing is considered to be *not* indicated for Wenckebach (Mobitz type I) A-V block associated with acute diaphragmatic MI in most cases. On the other hand, in many clinical situations, e.g., as in right BBB (RBBB) alone, left anterior or posterior hemiblock alone, and left BBB (LBBB) alone produced during acute MI, the true value of prophylactic pacing is still not yet certain, and there is significant disagreement among cardiologists.

The general trend in the use of artificial pacing has changed markedly in recent years, particularly in acute MI. For example, many patients who developed Wenckebach A-V block associated with acute diaphragmatic MI had been paced until 10 to 15 years ago. Now we no longer pace these patients because it became clear that Wenckebach A-V block in acute diaphragmatic MI is usually transient and no siginficant hemodynamic alterations are produced.

Current views regarding the indications and nonindications of temporary and permanent artificial pacemakers in acute MI are described in this chapter.

PATHOPHYSIOLOGICAL, CLINICAL, AND ECG CONSIDERATIONS

It is a well known fact that in nearly 90 to 95% of patients with acute MI some type of cardiac arrhythmia is observed, particularly during the first 72 hr of the illness. It is also well documented that every known cardiac arrhythmia can occur in patients with acute MI. Some cardiac arrhythmias, e.g., ventricular parasystole, nonparoxysmal ventricular (idioventricular) tachycardia (accelerated ventricular rhythm), and Wenckebach A-V block, are relatively benign and self-limited, whereas others, e.g., Mobitz type II A-V block, acute BFB or TFB, and paroxysmal ventricular tachycardia (VT), are potentially serious and require an active therapeutic approach.

In this section of the chapter, various cardiac rhythm disturbances in acute diaphragmatic MI versus anterior MI are compared in view of the indications or nonindications of artificial pacing in conjunction with the associated morbidity and mortality.

Incidence of Cardiac Arrhythmias

The incidence of various cardiac arrhythmias in acute diaphragmatic MI versus acute anterior MI is significantly different (Table 7-1).

1. For example, disturbances of sinus impulse formation and conduction, especially sinus bradycardia, are extremely common in acute diaphragmatic MI but are uncommon in acute anterior MI. The frequent occurrence of sick sinus syndrome (SSS) in acute diaphragmatic MI is emphasized elsewhere (see Chapter 4).

2. Similarly, nonparoxysmal A-V junctional tachycardia is nearly always found in acute diaphragmatic MI and not in acute anterior MI. At times, marked sinus bradycardia and nonparoxysmal A-V junctional tachycardia coexist with acute diaphragmatic MI.

TABLE 7-1. Incidence of Cardiac Arrhythmias in Diaphragmatic MI Versus Anterior MI

Arrhythmia	Diaphragmatic MI	Anterior MI
Sinus arrhythmias	Extremely common	Uncommon
Atrial arrhythmias	Uncommon	Uncommon
Nonparoxysmal A-V junctional tachycardia	Extremely common	Unusual
Ventricular arrhythmias	Extremely common	Extremely common
A-V block (all types)	Very common	Less common
Intraventricular blocks (all types)	Unusual	Extremely common
Parasystole	Rare	Rare

3. Conversely, various intraventricular blocks are almost always encountered in acute anterior MI as a result of permanent damage in the fascicles, but these conduction disturbances are extremely unusual in acute diaphragmatic MI.

4. A-V blocks (all types and degrees) are much more common in acute diaphragmatic MI than in anterior MI, but the outcome is benign in the former.

Incidence of A-V and Intraventricular Blocks

The incidence of various A-V conduction disturbances and intraventricular blocks in acute diaphragmatic MI versus anterior MI is summarized in Table 7-2.

1. Mobitz type II A-V block (see Figure 2-2) is usually encountered in acute anterior MI, whereas Wenckebach (Mobitz type I) A-V block is always found in acute diaphragmatic MI.

2. The 2:1 A-V block may be a variant of either Wenckebach A-V block or Mobitz type II A-V block.

3. In this circumstance, 2:1 A-V block is usually a variant of Wenckebach A-V block when the QRS complex is normal (narrow), especially during acute diaphragmatic MI.

4. In contrast, 2:1 A-V block is nearly always a variant of Mobitz type II A-V block when the QRS complex shows RBBB, LBBB, and BFB or incomplete TFB. Of course, definite differentiation between these A-V blocks can be accomplished by the His bundle electrocardiogram (ECG) (see Chapter 2).

General Features of Complete A-V Block

General features of complete A-V block in acute diaphragmatic MI versus acute anterior MI are summarized in Table 7-3.

1. The incidence of complete A-V block in acute diaphragmatic MI is about two to three times greater than that of acute anterior MI.

2. Yet the mortality is much higher (75%) in complete A-V block associated with anterior MI than that with diaphragmatic MI (only 20 to 40%). The reason for this finding is that the damage to the conduction system (infranodal block) in acute anterior MI is usually irreversible, and

TABLE 7-2. Incidence of A-V and Intraventricular Blocks in Diaphragmatic Versus Anterior MI

Block	Diaphragmatic MI	Anterior MI
First degree A-V block	Common	Rare
Wenckebach (Mobitz type I) A-V block	Extremely common	None
Mobitz type II A-V block	None	Common
2:1 A-V block	Variant of Wenckebach A-V block	Variant of Mobitz type II A-V block
Complete A-V block	A-V nodal block	Infranodal block
Intraventricular blocks (all types)	Unusual	Extremely common

TABLE 7-3. General Features of Complete A-V Block in Diaphragmatic MI Versus Anterior MI

Parameter	Diaphragmatic MI	Anterior MI
Incidence	More frequent (2–3 times)	Less frequent
Symptoms	Often asymptomatic	Often symptomatic
Damage to conduction tissue	Reversible	Irreversible
Duration	Usually transient	Usually permanent
Mortality	20–40%	More than 75%

there is a much higher incidence of other complications, e.g., CHF and cardiogenic shock. Thus temporary pacing followed by permanent pacemaker is definitely indicated under this circumstance.

3. On the other hand, complete A-V block (intranodal block) in acute diaphragmatic MI is usually reversible (because of ischemic change) and often asymptomatic. The cardiac pacing is *not* indicated in most cases with complete A-V block in acute diaphragmatic MI unless the ventricular rate is extremely slow (below 45 beats/min) and the patient is symptomatic (e.g., dizziness, hypotension, CHF, syncope).

ECG Findings of Complete A-V Block

As far as the ECG findings of complete A-V block in acute diaphragmatic MI versus anterior MI are concerned, significantly different features are observed (Table 7-4).

1. Because of the nature of intranodal block in acute diaphragmatic MI, the A-V junctional escape rhythm has a relatively stable and faster (45 to 60 beats/min) ventricular rate with normal (narrow) QRS complexes.

2. On the other hand, the ventricular escape (idioventricular) rhythm caused by infranodal block in anterior MI is often irregular and unstable with a slower ventricular rate (25 to 40 beats/min) and broad QRS complexes.

3. The His bundle ECG findings, of course, distinguish between A-V nodal block and infranodal block (see Chapter 2).

TABLE 7-4. ECG Findings of Complete A-V Block in Diaphragmatic MI Versus Anterior MI

Finding	Diaphragmatic MI	Anterior MI
Site of block	A-V nodal block	Infranodal block
His bundle ECG	A-deflection not followed by H-deflection	A-H deflections not followed by V-deflection
Escape rate	45–60	25–40
Origin of escape impulse	Lower A-V node (N-H region) or His bundle	Ventricles
Regularity of escape rhythm	Regular	May be irregular
QRS contour	Normal	Abnormal (wide)

FACTORS INFLUENCING INDICATIONS AND NONINDICATIONS FOR ARTIFICIAL PACING IN ACUTE MI

There are numerous factors which influence the indications and nonindications for artificial pacing in acute MI (Table 7-5).

Physician's Philosophy, Background, and Medical Knowledge

Each physician's philosophy, background, and medical knowledge as well as experience certainly influence the decision-making process.

1. For example, the physician with a conservative nature and one who is aggressive will have different attitudes toward the use of artificial pacing.

2. Another good example is that the physician with "up-to-date" medical knowledge will *not* use the artificial pacemakers for Wenckebach A-V block in acute diaphragmatic MI, whereas the physician with only old knowledge will use pacing in this case.

3. On the other hand, the His bundle electrophysiologists will frequently utilize the His bundle ECG results, e.g., the value of the H-V interval, to determine the indications versus nonindications for pacing in acute MI.

Presence or Absence of Symptoms

Needless to say, the most important factor is the presence or absence of symptoms (e.g., near-syncope, syncope, hypotension, heart failure) directly resulting from the conduction disturbances. Artificial pacing is indicated for all *symptomatic* arrhythmias, particularly high degree or complete A-V block, SSS, and BBBB (BFB and TFB).

Ventricular Rate

When the ventricular rate is slower than 40 beats/min, artificial pacing is indicated in acute MI because the patient is often symptomatic, and the extremely slow rhythm is potentially serious even if the patient is asymptomatic at the moment.

TABLE 7-5. Factors Influencing Indications Versus Nonindications for Artificial Pacing in Acute MI

1. Physician's philosophy, background, and medical knowledge
2. Presence or absence of symptoms
3. Ventricular rate
4. Location of myocardial infarction
5. Mechanism of arrhythmias, including type and location of heart blocks
6. Presence or absence of sick sinus syndrome and bradytachyarrhythmia syndrome
7. Availability of medical facilities and medical-surgical team for artificial pacing
8. Repose to antiarrhythmic drug therapy and direct current shock

Location of the MI

The location of the MI is, of course, a very important consideration. In general, artificial pacing is more frequently required for anterior MI than diaphragmatic MI.

Mechanisms of Arrhythmias

The mechanisms of the various arrhythmias and the site of the heart block definitely influence the use of pacing. For example, infranodal block always requires artificial pacing (usually a permanent unit), whereas an A-V nodal block (intranodal block) seldom necessitates the use of artificial pacing in acute MI.

Sick Sinus Syndrome

Artificial pacing is nearly always required for SSS and bradytachyarrhythmia syndrome (see Chapter 4).

Refractory Tachyarrhythmias

When any ectopic tachyarrhythmia—commonly paroxysmal VT or ventricular fibrillation (VF)—becomes refractory to common antiarrhythmic agents and/or direct current (DC) shock, the use of artificial pacing (overdrive pacing rate) should be considered regardless of the location of the MI.

Availability of Medical Facilities and Medical Team

One of the most important factors is, without a doubt, the availability of adequate medical facilities as well as the availability of medical-surgical teams who are capable of performing the artificial pacing procedures.

INDICATIONS FOR ARTIFICIAL PACING IN ACUTE MI REGARDLESS OF LOCATION

Indications of artificial pacing in acute MI regardless of its location are summarized in Table 7-6.

TABLE 7-6. Indications for Artificial Pacing in Acute MI Regardless of Location

1. Symptomatic and drug-resistant bradyarrhythmias of any origin or mechanism
   a. Sinus bradycardia, sinus arrest, S-A block
   b. A-V junctional and ventricular escape rhythm
   c. A-V block (second degree, high degree, and complete)
   d. Bilateral bundle branch block (bifascicular and trifascicular blocks)
2. Sick sinus syndrome and bradytachyarrhythmia syndrome
3. Drug-resistant ectopic tachyarrhythmias
4. Direct current shock-resistant tachyarrhythmias
5. Ventricular standstill

1. Artificial pacing is definitely indicated for all symptomatic and drug-resistant bradyarrhythmias, particularly high degree or complete A-V block and BFB or TFB (see Figure 2-5; see also Chapters 2 and 3).

2. For SSS and bradytachyarrhythmia syndrome, artificial pacing (often a permanent unit) is also indicated (see Figures 2-7 and 2-8; see also Chapter 4).

3. Drug-resistant and/or DC shock-resistant ectopic tachyarrhythmias likewise require artificial pacing with an overdriving rate.

4. Artificial pacing is indicated for ventricular standstill, but the outcome is very grave because of far-advanced underlying heart disease with irreversible other complications (e.g., cardiogenic shock).

INDICATIONS FOR ARTIFICIAL PACING IN ACUTE DIAPHRAGMATIC MI

As stressed previously, artificial pacing is required much less frequently in patients with acute diaphragmatic (inferior) MI than in those with anterior MI. Nevertheless, the pacing is definitely indicated in certain critical situations (Table 7-7).

1. The most important clinical circumstance which requires artificial pacing is drug-resistant symptomatic bradyarrhythmias, including second degree, high degree, or complete A-V block and sinus bradyarrhythmias.

2. In general, artificial pacing is indicated when the ventricular rate is slower than 40 beats/min, particularly in high degree (advanced) or complete A-V block in acute diaphragmatic MI.

3. Wenckebach A-V block may coexist with Wenckebach S-A block in which pacing is indicated when the heart block is symptomatic and/or the ventricular rate is below 40 beats/min.

4. In addition, artificial pacing is indicated for SSS, bradytachyarrhythmia syndrome, refractory ectopic tachyarrhythmias, and ventricular standstill.

5. Artificial pacing is *not* indicated for first degree A-V block or Wenckebach (Mobitz type I) A-V block unless the patient is symptomatic and/or the ventricular rate is very slow (below 40 beats/min).

Indications for Artificial Pacing in Acute Anterior MI

Although the incidence of A-V block is much less common in acute anterior MI than in acute diaphragmatic MI (Tables 7-1 to 7-4), artificial

TABLE 7-7. Indications of Artificial Pacing in Acute Diaphragmatic MI

1. Drug-resistant symptomatic second degree, high degree, or complete A-V block; sinus bradycardia; sinus arrest; S-A block; A-V junctional escape rhythm
2. Extremely slow ventricular rate (below 45 beats/min) due to any mechanism
3. Sick sinus syndrome and bradytachyarrhythmia syndrome
4. Refractory ectopic tachyarrhythmias
5. Ventricular standstill

TABLE 7-8. Indications for Artificial Pacing in Acute Anterior MI

1. Complete A-V block: pacing (often permanent) in every case regardless of symptoms
2. Mobitz type II A-V block
3. Drug-resistant symptomatic sinus bradycardia, sinus arrest, S-A block, slow escape rhythm without A-V block
4. Sick sinus syndrome and bradytachyarrhythmia syndrome
5. Various forms of bilateral bundle branch block (bifascicular and trifascicular block) with acute onset
6. Refractory ectopic tachyarrhythmias
7. Ventricular standstill

pacing is almost always required once the patient develops A-V block in the former. The reason for this is that the block is the end result of permanent damage in the fascicles (infranodal block) in most cases of anterior MI. For the same reason, various forms of intraventricular blocks are commonly observed in acute anterior MI. Table 7-8 summarizes the indications of artificial pacing in acute anterior MI.

1. Complete A-V block in acute anterior MI represents complete infranodal block (complete TFB), which usually requires permanent pacing.

2. For a similar reason, pacing is indicated in patients who develop Mobitz type II A-V block as a result of acute anterior MI (see Figure 2-2) regardless of symptoms because Mobitz type II A-V block represents incomplete infranodal block and is a precursor of complete A-V block—complete TFB.

3. Prophylactic artificial pacing is recommended for all forms of acute incomplete bilateral bundle branch block (BBBB).

4. For example, prophylactic pacing is indicated for a BFB which consists of RBBB and left anterior or posterior hemiblock with or without first degree A-V block (see Figure 2-5). A combination of RBBB and left anterior hemiblock is the most common bifascicular block in acute anterior MI (see Figure 2-5) and carries a mortality of approximately 40% in most reports.

5. On the other hand, a BFB consisting of RBBB and left posterior hemiblock is much less common, comprising no more than 10% of all BFBs in acute MI. Yet it is reported to be associated with a mortality rate of more than 80% in some studies.

6. Under these circumstances, prophylactic pacing is more urgently needed when there is marked first degree A-V block (P-R interval: 0.28 sec or more), when RBBB and LBBB occur alternately, or when left anterior and posterior hemiblock occur on different occasions in the presence of acute RBBB.

7. For acute LBBB, RBBB, or left posterior hemiblock with or without first degree A-V block in acute anterior MI, the use of prophylactic artificial pacing is *not* uniformly agreed on (discussed later in the chapter).

NO VALUE OF ARTIFICIAL PACING IN ACUTE MI

In certain clinical situations, it is clear that artificial pacing provides no benefit in acute MI (Table 7-9).

1. For example, first degree A-V block or Wenckebach A-V block is extremely common in the early phase of acute diaphragmatic MI, but no pacing is indicated in these circumstances unless the ventricular rate is very slow (below 40 beats/min) and/or the patient is symptomatic.

2. Similarly, no pacing is indicated for asymptomatic or transient sinus or A-V junctional bradyarrhythmias, which are common in acute diaphragmatic MI.

3. Nonparoxysmal A-V junctional or ventricular tachycardia or ventricular parasystolic tachycardia is usually self-limited, and no pacing is required for these arrhythmias.

4. Isolated left anterior hemiblock is the most common fascicular block in patients with acute MI, being encountered in 15% of all MI patients. Left anterior hemiblock is much more common in acute anterior MI than in diaphragmatic MI. However, less than 10% of patients with left anterior hemiblock in anterior MI may develop advanced fascicular blocks, e.g., bifascicular or trifascicular block. At any rate, prophylactic pacing is *not* indicated for isolated left anterior hemiblock (either acute or preexisting) in acute MI.

5. In addition, prophylactic pacing is *not* required for preexisting isolated RBBB, LBBB, or left posterior hemiblock in acute MI.

6. When these fascicular blocks occur acutely as a result of acute MI, the therapeutic approach is different (see below).

EQUIVOCAL OR QUESTIONABLE VALUE OF ARTIFICIAL PACING IN ACUTE MI

A profound controversy exists among physicians regarding the use of artificial pacemakers in acute MI in certain clinical situations (Table 7-10). In other words, it is not certain if the pacing is indicated because the value of prophylactic pacing is equivocal.

1. For example, some cardiologists recommend prophylactic pacing for acute isolated RBBB, LBBB, or left posterior hemiblock in acute MI. In these circumstances, the value of prophylactic pacing is probably

TABLE 7-9. No Value of Artificial Pacing in Acute MI

1. First degree A-V block alone (acute or preexisting)
2. Asymptomatic Wenckebach A-V block (acute or preexisting)
3. Asymptomatic or transient sinus or A-V junctional bradyarrhythmias
4. Nonparoxysmal A-V junctional or ventricular tachycardia and ventricular parasystolic tachycardia
5. Left anterior hemiblock alone (acute or preexisting)
6. Preexisting right or left bundle branch block alone, or left posterior hemiblock alone

TABLE 7-10. Equivocal or Questionable Value of Artificial Pacing in Acute MI

1. Acute right bundle branch block alone
2. Acute left bundle branch block alone
3. Acute left posterior hemiblock alone
4. Transient acute bifascicular block (asymptomatic)
5. Acute left or right bundle branch block or left anterior or posterior hemiblock with first degree A-V block and/or prolonged H-V interval
6. Late (more than 1 week after the onset of the acute episode) development of acute bifascicular block (asymptomatic)
7. Preexisting bifascicular or incomplete trifascicular block (asymptomatic)

greater for acute LBBB or left posterior hemiblock than for acute RBBB in acute MI.

2. Isolated RBBB occurs in 1 to 7% of all MI patients. Overall mortality in some series is reported to be 40%, and it may be as high as 74%.

3. Isolated acute LBBB is encountered in 4 to 6% of acute MI patients, and the mortality is about 35 to 50%. Although it is often uncertain when LBBB is a preexisting abnormality or when it is the direct result of acute MI, prophylactic pacing is frequently recommended when the duration of LBBB is not definitely known.

4. Isolated acute left posterior hemiblock is an uncommon fascicular block in acute MI, but the prophylactic pacing is usually recommended because it is shown to commonly progress to higher degree fascicular blocks, e.g., BFB or TFB.

5. When acute LBBB, RBBB, or left anterior or posterior hemiblock is associated with first degree A-V block and/or a prolonged H-V interval, prophylactic pacing is highly recommended because this group is at high risk of abrupt progression to advanced or complete A-V block (complete TFB).

6. The true value of prophylactic pacing for preexisting BFB or incomplete TFB (asymptomatic) in acute MI is uncertain.

7. In addition, the value of the pacing for transient acute BFB (asymptomatic) or late development of acute BFB (asymptomatic) in acute MI is also unclear. Nevertheless, some physicians recommend prophylactic pacing for these groups.

INDICATIONS FOR PERMANENT ARTIFICIAL PACING IN ACUTE MI

It is immensely important to determine if permanent pacing is definitely indicated in patients with acute MI associated with various cardiac arrhythmias because in many cases the pacing may be the only lifesaving measure. Generally acceptable criteria for indications of permanent artificial pacing in acute MI are summarized in Table 7-11.

1. Unquestionably, permanent pacing is indicated for all patients who develop Mobitz type II A-V block or complete A-V block (complete TFB) in acute anterior MI regardless of symptom.

TABLE 7-11. Indications for Permanent Artificial Pacing in Acute MI

1. Mobitz type II A-V block regardless of symptoms
2. Complete A-V block (complete trifascicular block—infranodal block) in acute anterior myocardial infarction regardless of symptoms
3. Sick sinus syndrome and bradytachyarrhythmia syndrome regardless of location of myocardial infarction
4. Symptomatic and drug-resistant bradyarrhythmias with very slow ventricular rate (below 45 beats/min) in acute diaphragmatic myocardial infarction lasting more than 2–3 weeks
5. Persisting drug-resistant and/or DC-shock-resistant ectopic tachyarrhythmias benefited by temporary pacing
6. Acute bifascicular block with intermittent complete A-V block (incomplete trifascicular block) in acute anterior myocardial infarction regardless of symptoms
7. All incomplete trifascicular blocks

2. Permanent pacing is also indicated for SSS (see Chapter 4) and bradytachyarrhythmia syndrome (see Figures 2-7 and 2-8).

3. When symptomatic bradyarrhythmias, particularly high degree or complete A-V block (usually very slow ventricular rate) persist more than 2 to 3 weeks in acute diaphragmatic MI, permanent pacing should be considered.

4. Permanent pacing is occasionally indicated for persisting drug-resistant and/or DC shock-resistant ectopic tachyarrhythmias (usually ventricular tachyarrhythmias) benefited by temporary pacing (see Chapter 5).

5. Recently, it has been shown that there is high incidence of sudden death in patients with acute anterior MI associated with acute BFB and intermittent complete A-V block within 6 months after discharge from the hospital. Thus permanent pacing is recommended for this group of high risk patients.

6. Although it is not uniformly agreed on, many cardiologists recommend permanent pacing for all forms of acute incomplete TFB in acute MI regardless of symptom. Incomplete TFB may include BFB (a combination of RBBB and left anterior or posterior hemiblock) plus first degree A-V block and/or a prolonged H-V interval, alternating LBBB and RBBB, and RBBB with left anterior hemiblock on one occasion and RBBB with left posterior hemiblock on another occasion with or without first degree A-V block.

7. Some physicians also recommend permanent pacing for acute LBBB with first degree A-V block and for acute RBBB with left posterior hemiblock alone in acute MI, but this view is not accepted by others.

Detailed descriptions regarding various indications of permanent pacing are found in Chapter 8.

Permanent Pacing: Indications

8

The decision about whether to institute permanent cardiac pacing should be made with extreme caution. The reason for this is, obviously, that once the pacemaker is implanted it is difficutlt to remove. Moreover, the daily care with its associated precautions related to artificial pacemakers should be followed in persons with permanent pacemakers as well, and reliable follow-up care by the physician who is fully familiar with the pacemaker is mandatory (see Chapters 1 and 12). Finally, the pulse generator must be replaced every 10 to 12 years (every 3 to 6 years for older models) to avoid the development of malfunctions.

There is always a potential danger of the pacemaker developing a malfunction. Therefore it is not advisable for any individual with a permanent pacemaker to travel to any part of the world where adequate medical-surgical facilities with well trained personnel are not available.

In addition to the medical aspects, the legal considerations relating to permanent artificial pacing are important.

Permanent pacemakers must not be over- or underused. In most clinical situations, the cardiologist has the main role in determining the indications versus the nonindications for permanent pacing. The cardiac surgeon usually relies on the opinion of the cardiologist before implanting a permanent pacemaker.

Indications for permanent pacemaker implantation have changed during the past several years. Until a few years ago, the main indication for permanent pacing was for complete atrioventricular (A-V) block. The recent trend, however, has been more frequent usage of permanent pacing for sick sinus syndrome (SSS) (see Chapter 4). It can be said with reasonable certainty that the most common indication for permanent pacemaker implantation today is for the management of patients with SSS, in whom various conduction disturbances coexist, including A-V and/or fascicular blocks (see Chapter 4).

When the indication for a permanent pacemaker has been determined, the type and the mode of pacemaker most suitable for a given individual must be chosen taking into consideration the patient's age, general condition, and underlying heart disease, as well as the mechanism of the cardiac arrhythmia(s). In most clinical situations, particularly in older individuals, a conventional ventricular demand pacemaker is adequate for ordinary daily activity. On the other hand, the general trend today is to use multiprogrammable pacemakers in a variety of clinical circumstances so that various pacemaker functions can be adjusted, when necessary, after implantation.

When the atrial contribution (kick) is definitely necessary to improve cardiac output in patients with advanced heart disease, ventricular pacing is not ideal. A fixed-rate ventricular pacemaker must be avoided when intermittent restoration of the patient's own natural rhythm is expected, as in intermittent A-V block and incomplete bilateral bundle branch block (BBBB) (see Chapters 2 and 3). Otherwise, competition between the natural rhythm and the artificial pacemaker rhythm may cause ventricular fibrillation and even sudden death as a result of the R-on-T phenomenon (see Chapters 1 and 12).

Although there are slightly different views among physicians, in the following clinical situations permanent (long-term) pacing is considered to be indicated (Table 8-1).

Sick Sinus Syndrome and Bradytachyarrhythmia Syndrome

As emphasized repeatedly, the most common indication for permanent cardiac pacing today is for the management of SSS. Drug therapy is totally ineffective for this syndrome.

1. Permanent pacing is indicated in all patients with symptomatic (e.g., dizziness, near-syncope, or actual syncope) and advanced SSS.
2. The most common manifestation of SSS is marked sinus bradycardia, which is frequently associated with intermittent sinus arrest or sinoatrial (S-A) block and areas of A-V junctional escape rhythm (see Figures 4-1 and 4-3).
3. In more advanced forms of SSS, chronic atrial fibrillation or

TABLE 8-1. Indications for Permanent Pacing

1. Sick sinus syndrome and bradytachyarrhythmia syndrome
2. Mobitz type II A-V block
3. Complete or advanced A-V block
   a. Caused by trifascicular block
   b. Congenital
   c. Surgically induced (irreversible)
   d. Lasting more than 2–3 weeks in acute myocardial infarction
   e. All other chronic and symptomatic A-V blocks
4. Symptomatic bilateral bundle branch blocks
5. Bifascicular block or incomplete trifascicular block with intermittent complete A-V block as a result of acute myocardial infarction
6. Carotid sinus syncope
7. Recurrent ventricular standstill
8. Recurrent drug-resistant tachyarrhythmias benefited by temporary pacing

flutter is the end result, and there is usually a slow ventricular rate caused by advanced A-V block (see Figure 4-6).

4. When SSS is far advanced, various tachyarrhythmia components—e.g., ventricular premature contractions (VPCs), ventricular group beats or tachycardia, and various atrial tachyarrhythmias—develop and the resulting rhythm abnormality is bradytachyarrhythmia syndrome (see Figures 1-6, 4-2, and 4-3). Hence bradytachyarrhythmia is a common end result of the late stage of far-advanced SSS.

5. In most situations, an ordinary ventricular demand pacemaker is adequate for the management of SSS, but ideal pacing is carried out by the multiprogrammable pacemakers.

6. When the atrial contribution (kick) is critically needed to improve cardiac output, atrial pacing, e.g., coronary sinus pacing, may be beneficial. A main advantage of using atrial pacing is that the atrial tachyarrhythmia component may be suppressed by this mode of pacing.

7. Atrial-synchronized or bifocal demand pacing should be used for patients with SSS associated with A-V block when the atrial contribution is definitely required.

8. In bradytachyarrhythmia syndrome, one or more antiarrhythmic agents—e.g., quinidine, procainamide, disopyramide phosphate (Norpace), propranolol, and digitalis may be required when the tachyarrhythmia component persists even after permanent pacemaker implantation.

SSS is discussed in detail in Chapter 4.

Mobitz Type II A-V Block

1. Permanent pacing is indicated for all patients with Mobitz type II A-V block (see Figure 2-2) regardless of whether the patient is symptomatic because Mobitz type II A-V block represents infranodal block, which is irreversible (see Chapter 2).

2. Mobitz type II A-V block frequently leads to advanced A-V block [incomplete trifascicular block (TFB); see Figure 3-3], and it is often a precursor of complete A-V (infranodal) block caused by complete TFB (see Figure 2-6).

3. A variant of Mobitz type II A-V block is often manifested by 2:1 A-V block in which the QRS morphology almost always exhibits RBBB or LBBB, hemiblocks, bifascicular block (BFB), or incomplete TFB (see Figure 2-3).

Mobitz type II A-V block is described in detail in Chapter 2.

Complete or Advanced A-V Block

Factors for determining indications of permanent pacing in advanced or complete A-V block include the site of the block, the presence or absence of symptoms (e.g., near-syncope or syncope), the ventricular rate, the duration of the A-V block, and the underlying disease processes.

1. Permanent pacing is indicated for all patients with advanced or complete A-V block as a result of TFB (see Figures 2-6 and 3-3). In these circumstances, the patient is symptomatic in nearly all cases.

2. When the QRS complex is normal (narrow) and the ventricular rate is very slow (below 40 beats/min) in complete A-V block, the site of the block is considered to be in the His bundle. Complete His bundle block is also an infranodal block, which is treated the same way as complete TFB. Permanent pacing is indicated in this case.

3. When complete A-V block is produced after major cardiac surgery and when it lasts more than 1 week, irreversible damage in the A-V conduction system is considered to be present. Thus permanent pacing is recommended for most patients with surgically induced chronic complete A-V block.

4. The fact that there is a marked discrepancy regarding the nature, underlying mechanism, symptomatology, outcome, etc. of complete A-V block in anterior versus diaphragmatic MI has been emphasized (see Chapter 7).

5. Permanent pacing (after temporary pacing) is indicated in almost all patients with complete A-V block in acute anterior MI because the block is irreversible.

6. On the other hand, artificial pacing is unlikely to be indicated for complete A-V block in diaphragmatic MI unless the ventricular rate is slower than 40 beats/min and/or the patient is symptomatic.

7. Nevertheless, permanent pacing is recommended for all patients who suffer from acute MI when complete A-V block lasts more than 2 to 3 weeks.

8. By and large, permanent pacing is indicated for all patients with chronic complete A-V block, particularly when the patient is symptomatic regardless of the clinical circumstances.

9. All patients with congenital complete A-V block eventually require permanent pacing regardless of whether there is a coexisting congenital cardiac defect, although some individuals may be totally asymptomatic in spite of complete A-V block.

Symptomatic Bilateral Bundle Branch Block

BBBBs include BFB and TFB (see Chapter 3).

1. When BBBB is said to be symptomatic (e.g., dizziness, near-syncope, or syncope), there is intermittent occurrence of bradyarrhythmias—areas of advanced or complete TFB (see Figure 3-3).

2. Needless to say, complete A-V block is the resulting abnormality when there is complete TFB (see Figure 2-6).

3. In many cases the patient develops various forms of BFB or incomplete TFB before the occurrence of advanced or complete A-V block.

4. The initial electrocardiographic (ECG) findings may consist of RBBB and left posterior hemiblock with or without first degree A-V block (the P-R interval: often 0.28 sec or more; see Figure 3-2).

5. On other occasions the same patient may develop another form of incomplete BBBB which consists of RBBB and left anterior hemiblock with or without first degree A-V block.

6. Many cardiologists recommend prophylactic permanent pacing when the ECG findings exhibit BFB with marked first degree A-V block (P-R interval: 0.28 sec or more) and/or a prolonged H-V interval (70 msec or more), even before the actual development of advanced or complete A-V block.

7. When there are documented episodes of advanced or complete A-V block in patients with incomplete BBBB, implantation of a permanent pacemaker is relatively urgent. In this circumstance temporary pacing should be carried out before permanent pacemaker implantation when the patient is symptomatic and/or the ventricular rate is markedly slow (less than 40 beats/min).

BFB or Incomplete TFB with Intermittent Complete A-V Block Resulting from Acute MI

It was recently shown that the potential risk of sudden death is great within 6 months of an acute MI when BFB or incomplete TFB is associated with intermittent complete A-V block during infarction. Thus a permanent pacemaker is recommended for every patient in this circumstance before discharge from the hospital (see Chapter 7).

Carotid Sinus Syncope

A permanent pacemaker is unequivocally indicated in all patients with carotid sinus syncope (see Figure 4-8). When the patient shows significant symptoms (e.g., near-syncope or syncope), temporary pacing may be carried out before the implantation of a permanent pacemaker. Carotid sinus syncope is often a manifestation of SSS (see Chapter 4).

Recurrent Ventricular Standstill

When ventricular standstill recurs chronically, regardless of the underlying mechanism or disease process, permanent pacing is indicated, particularly when the patient is symptomatic. Of course, the underlying process responsible for the production of ventricular standstill may be SSS and/or carotid sinus syncope, but in some cases no clear etiological factor can be found.

Recurrent Drug-Resistant Tachyarrhythmias Benefited by Temporary Pacing

When refractory ectopic tachyarrhythmias, particularly paroxysmal VT recur as soon as the temporary pacing is turned off, permanent pacing should be considered. Suitable pacing rate should be determined during temporary pacing on an individual basis. In most situations, an overdriving pacing rate (rate: 80 to 120 beats/min) is necessary to suppress refractory tachyarrhythmias.

Artificial Pacing: Modifying Factors

9

FACTORS MODIFYING THE PACING STIMULATORY THRESHOLD

Effective pacemaker function depends on the physiological, pathophysiological, and pharmacological environment at the pacemaker electrode tip-myocardial interface. If the electrophysiological properties of myocardial threshold, conductivity, or refractoriness are affected adversely, an otherwise normally functioning pacemaker may be unable to stimulate the myocardium. This situation is often termed pacemaker exit block. Stimulatory threshold—defined as the minimal electrical impulse necessary to stimulate the heart for the electrical system used—best reflects these electrophysiological variables. The threshold is not static, and multiple factors have been demonstrated to cause fluctuations in the threshold value. The following review discusses those factors which are clinically pertinent. Factors which may reduce or increase the myocardial threshold are summarized in Tables 9-1 and 9-2.

PHYSIOLOGICAL VARIABLES

Physiological variables in the patient's daily routine activity may affect stimulatory threshold (Tables 9-1 and 9-2).

1. Orthostatic conditions alone usually result in a 5 to 10% reduction of the threshold. It has been demonstrated that the threshold is 10 to 25% higher in the resting than in the active state, with a 30 to 40% increase in the threshold during sleep.
2. Submaximal stress can decrease stimulatory threshold by as much as 30% over baseline values.
3. Bradyarrhythmias caused by a malfunctioning pacemaker during sleep have been documented to correct spontaneously with resumption of the wakeful state and activity.
4. Eating is another common variable that affects stimulatory

TABLE 9-1. Factors with a Tendency to Reduce the Myocardial Threshold

1. Exercise and orthostatic state
2. Acute elevation of serum potassium
3. Sympathomimetic stimulation
4. Glucocorticoids
5. Aldosterone antagonists
6. Digitalis (?)

threshold. The glucose load associated with meals has been shown to result in a 30% increase in threshold. This effect is related to changes in the intracellular potassium concentration and is described in more detail later in the chapter. The same phenomenon explains why wide fluctuations in blood glucose in the diabetic patient may result in transient pacemaker malfunction.

INFLAMMATORY AND INFECTIVE PROCESSES

1. After implantation, pacemaker stimulatory threshold normally rises and reaches a maximum at 5 to 10 days.
2. This initial rise is followed by a gradual decline in threshold, with stabilization by approximately 3 weeks.
3. The maximal stimulatory threshold usually does not exceed two to three times the initial value.
4. This phenomenon is thought to be secondary to both microdislocations at the pacemaker electrode tip and local tissue reaction at the endocardial contact point.
5. Any superimposed inflammatory or infective process (e.g., myocarditis or endocarditis) would be expected to exaggerate this foreign body response and cause an abnormal elevation of threshold (Table 9-2).

BLOOD GAS AND ACID-BASE ABNORMALITIES

The interplay of blood-gas and acid-base abnormalities is complex, and the net result in the individual patient may be difficult to predict (Table 9-2).

TABLE 9-2. Factors with a Tendency to Increase the Myocardial Threshold

1. Inflammation or infection at the pacemaker electrode tip
2. Sleep and resting state
3. Eating (glucose-insulin infusion)
4. Marked hyperkalemia or hypokalemia
5. Acute reduction of serum potassium
6. Elevation of serum sodium
7. Acidosis, alkalosis
8. Hypoxia, hypercarbia
9. Mineralocorticoids
10. Propranolol (Inderal) and other beta-adrenergic blocking agents
11. Procainamide (Pronestyl)
12. Quinidine (?)

Acidosis and Alkalosis

1. Both acidosis and alkalosis have been reported to result in a marked elevation of the stimulatory threshold.

2. This has clinical relevance in cases of cardiac resuscitation, in which large amounts of bicarbonate are frequently used.

3. It seems likely that bicarbonate therapy does not adversely affect pacemaker function when life-threatening situations require immediate treatment in the patient with an artificial pacemaker.

Hypoxia and Hypercarbia

1. Hypoxia increases the stimulatory threshold.

2. Coexisting acidosis tends to return the threshold toward normal.

3. It has been demonstrated that reducing the oxygen tension in blood by 42 mm Hg increases the stimulatory threshold from 3.4 to 5.7 volts and elevating the oxygen tension by 33 mm Hg reduces the stimulatory threshold from 3.4 to 2.6 volts.

4. Hypercarbia, with or without hypoxia, results in a marked increment of the stimulatory threshold, and hypocarbia results in its reduction.

5. Rapid changes in oxygen and carbon dioxide tension may occur clinically during the induction of general anesthesia, and adequate oxygenation and ventilation for the patient with a pacemaker must be guaranteed in this setting.

ELECTROLYTE ABNORMALITIES

Various electrolyte abnormalities may affect the pacing stimulatory threshold (Tables 9-1 and 9-2).

Potassium

1. Potassium fluctuations are the most significant of the electrolyte abnormalities that affect the stimulatory threshold.

2. Both hyper- and hypokalemia have been reported to be associated with transient pacemaker malfunction.

3. The absolute potassium level is not as critical as the intracellular/extracellular potassium concentration ratio.

4. An increase in extracellular potassium results in a reduction of membrane potential and an increase in electrical excitability.

5. Thus any intervention which reduces intracellular potassium in relation to extracellular potassium results in a reduction of stimulatory threshold, whereas the threshold rises when the intracellular/extracellular potassium ratio increases.

6. Intravenous potassium infusions which acutely increase serum potassium levels, so long as hyperkalemia is not produced, consistently reduce the threshold value.

7. Acute reduction of serum potassium (e.g., by glucose-insulin infusions) consistently elevates the threshold value.

8. By and large, failure of cardiac capture by an artificial pacemaker stimulus is most commonly secondary to severe hyperkalemia.

Sodium

1. Elevation of the extracellular sodium concentration results in an increase in membrane potential and a decrease in electrical excitability.
2. Intravenous infusions of sodium chloride generally result in an increase in the threshold.
3. The sodium retention and potassium loss induced by the mineralocorticoids result in an increase in the stimulatory threshold.
4. Spironolactone, an aldosterone antagonist, would be expected to reduce the stimulatory threshold by a similar mechanism.

Calcium

Intravenous calcium infusions in therapeutic doses have no demonstrable effect on the pacing stimulatory threshold.

DRUG EFFECTS

Various drugs have been demonstrated to affect the pacing stimulatory threshold (Tables 9-1 and 9-2).

Sympathomimetic Agents

Sympathomimetic agents increase myocardial excitability and reduce the threshold.

1. *Ephedrine sulfate* in doses of 25 mg every 6 hr reduces the threshold by 20%.
2. *Isoproterenol* (Isuprel) has been reported to restore pacing in patients with premature pacemaker failure, and *metaproterenol sulfate* (Alupent) has also been shown to lead to a short-term reduction of the stimulatory threshold.
3. *Propranolol* (Inderal) and other beta-adrenergic blocking agents block the increased myocardial excitability effect of the sympathomimetic drugs.

Antiarrhythmic Agents

The effects of the various antiarrhythmic agents on pacing stimulatory threshold are extremely important clinically.

1. *Propranolol* (Inderal) and other beta-adrenergic blocking agents increase the threshold, the effect proportional to the existing level of sympathetic tone.
2. Propranolol increases the threshold in patients who have been physically active and who have a high level of sympathetic activity, whereas no appreciable effect is noted in patients who have been in the resting state.
3. *Verapamil* is thought to have an effect similar to that of propranolol.
4. *Procainamide* (Pronestyl) in therapeutic doses results in a 10 to 15% elevation of the pacing stimulatory threshold. At toxic levels, procainamide has been documented to cause pacemaker failure in both capture and sensing functions.
5. There is little information in the literature concerning the effect of *quinidine,* but it would be anticipated to be similar to that of procainamide because of the similar pharmacology of the two drugs.

6. *Lidocaine* (Xylocaine) and *phenytoin* (Dilantin) probably have no significant effect on the pacing stimulatory threshold.

Digitalis

Digitalis has several important effects in the patient with an artificial pacemaker, but its effect on the pacing stimulatory threshold remains somewhat contradictory.

1. It has been shown that administration of digitalis increases minute and stroke volumes in patients with artificial pacemakers.
2. Theoretically, digitalis should decrease the threshold because of its known action of sensitizing the myocardium to ectopic stimuli.
3. It has been demonstrated that acute digitalization results in a significant reduction of the stimulatory threshold, from 2.8 to 2.1 volts.
4. Clinically, the effect of digitalis on the pacing stimulatory threshold does not seem to be significant.
5. Digitalis is definitely effective in patients with congestive heart failure (CHF) who have an artificial pacemaker.
6. It should be emphasized that the patient with an artificial pacemaker is *not* immune to digitalis toxicity (see Chapter 10).

Steroids

Glucocorticoids, in contrast to the mineralocorticoids, have been shown to consistently reduce the pacing stimulatory threshold, in part because they alter cellular membrane permeability. Therapeutically, glucocorticoids are commonly used in the treatment of "pacemaker exit block."

Miscellaneous

Acetylcholine does not affect the pacing stimulatory threshold and may be used without risk in patients with artificial pacemakers. Alcohol administration has also been shown to have no effect on the stimulatory threshold, and moderate alcohol consumption is thought to have no adverse effect on pacemaker function.

INTERFERENCES OF ARTIFICIAL CARDIAC PACING

Since the introduction of the artificial cardiac pacemaker into clinical medicine 20 years ago, the instrument has undergone considerable modification. It began as an instrument that emitted an electrical signal of given intensity at a given time frequency. Initially available only as an external device, internal implantation and synchronous circuitry were developed and various types of electrodes created.

From the beginning, however, artificial pacemakers have been plagued by the possibility of physical interference. With the increasing complexity of the instrument and electrical circuitry, it has become more vulnerable to new and different types of interference. At the same time, manufacturers have steadily been at work in an attempt to yield their equipment free from these effects. The pacemakers have been greatly improved in this regard, but up to the present time no pacemaker manufacturer has been completely successful in shielding instruments from physical interference.

Electromagnetic fields represent the only significant physical interference to which pacemakers are subjected. Because of the complexity and socioeconomics of modern society, it is extremely unlikely that sources of this interference can be completely eliminated or even decreased in the foreseeable future. Thus it seems that a working knowledge of what constitutes such interference and how to minimize it will enable the physician to maintain a healthy vigilance for the interferences and make proper recommendations to patients with artificial pacemakers.

CARDIAC PACEMAKERS AND ELECTRODES AND THEIR SUSCEPTIBILITIES

1. Artificial pacemakers may be external or internal, synchronous or asynchronous, and bipolar or unipolar. Each of these specifications predisposes the instrument to certain types of interference and may lead to different types of abnormal function. It is important to look at each characteristic individually in order to understand the susceptibility it produces.

2. The exposed position of external pacemakers versus internal pacemakers obviously subjects them to greater hazard, not only from electromagnetic interference but from more direct injurious stimuli (e.g., mechanical or water damage). It also creates the opportunity for small current leaks to the myocardium, leading to the development of ventricular fibrillation (VF). Meticulous care and adequate insulation of the pulse generator are mandatory.

3. Electromagnetic fields diminish rapidly as the distance from their source increases. Proximity is therefore of great importance in this regard. This factor is of more importance with external pacemakers and accounts for their enhanced susceptibility.

4. Originally, all artificial pacemakers were asynchronous and contained only a pacing circuit with a low frequency oscillator whose rate could be dramatically increased when exposed to high frequency interference. This, in turn, greatly increased the pacing rate of firing and produced rapid tachycardia or even VF. They were also susceptible to sudden severe electrical discharges, e.g., those produced by alternating current defibrillators. As pacemaker manufacturers became aware of these problems, the circuitry and shielding were modified. At approximately the same time these developments were taking place, the danger of producing VF by asynchronous pacing was being increasingly recognized, particularly in the presence of myocardial ischemia, and synchronous pacemakers were being developed.

5. Synchronous artificial pacemakers consist of two circuits, one for pacing and the other for sensing. The latter is designed to recognize intrinsic or spontaneous cardiac depolarization and to recycle the pacing circuit, thus preventing competition between the intrinsic rhythm and the pacing rhythm or the possibility of a pacer discharge occurring during the vulnerable period (R-on-T phenomenon). One of the problems created by such instruments is their inability to discriminate absolutely between the QRS complex (or P wave in atrial synchronous instruments) and extraneous electromagnetic interference.

6. Both the amplitude and the wave form of the sensed impulse are utilized for discrimination, but it is still not possible to avoid all electromagnetic interference. In response to this problem, many manufacturers have designed their instruments to revert to asynchronous function when overloaded by electromagnetic interference. This does not completely solve the problem, however, because some electromagnetic energy sources are noncontinuous and result in dangerous intermittent pauses rather than reversion to a fixed rate.

7. Pacemaker electrodes are either bipolar or unipolar. In the former, both cathode and anode are in contact with the myocardium, whereas in the latter the cathode is usually in contact with the myocardium and the anode is implanted subcutaneously at a more remote site.

8. Sensitivity to electromagnetic interference is proportionate to the distance between the cathode and the anode, which of course is much larger in the unipolar system.

9. The advantage of unipolar systems is that they have a superior sensing function. The number of such implants is currently increasing.

TYPES OF INTERFERENCE

All currently known significant external interferences for cardiac pacemakers are electromagnetic in nature (Tables 9-3 through 9-5).

TABLE 9-3. Electromagnetic Sources Unlikely to Interfere with Pacemaker Function

Household appliances
Small electric shop tools
Weapons detectors
Microwave ovens (shielded pacemakers)
Automatic switching devices
Smooth commutator motors
Dental equipment
Television and radio receivers

TABLE 9-4. Potential Sources of Electromagnetic Interference for Pacemakers

Defibrillators
Theft detectors
Ignition systems

TABLE 9-5. Electromagnetic Sources Likely to Interfere with Pacemaker Function

Diathermy equipment
Electric arc welders
Electrosurgical equipment
Radar installations
Ultrasonic cleaners

1. There is interference in varying degrees by virtually all electrical devices, ranging from ordinary household appliances to the largest equipment of heavy industry.

2. The interference is characterized by its frequency or the number of cycles it alternates each second.

3. Each source of interference must be tested against artificial pacemakers to determine the presence or absence of effect, the degree of such effect, and the pacemaker response.

4. The distributor and spark plugs of an automobile may accelerate the pacemaker discharge to 450 beats/min and cause a 7- to 10-sec delay in pacing when removed.

5. Similar deleterious effects secondary to a diathermy machine have been reported.

6. Alternating (AC) or direct (DC) current defibrillators may cause malfunction of the pacemaker.

7. Interference may be caused by surgical electrocautery, short wave diathermy, ultraviolet light machines, neon signs, radio transmitters, betatron therapy units, and other high-tension currents. When examined, the cause of the problem in these cases was considered to be high frequency oscillation induced in the pacemaker, and it was suggested that a circuit be designed to prevent it. Newer pacemakers no longer suffer from these difficulties.

8. The synchronous units may show greater variation. Some may become inactive, whereas others may revert to a fixed-rate operation or a maximum synchronous pacing rate.

9. Electrocautery continues to be one of the most hazardous iatrogenic stimuli despite the demonstration that proper shielding, grounding, and placement can help prevent this problem. Although most modern demand pacemakers revert to the asynchronous mode when exposed to electrocautery, care must be taken to avoid long periods of asystole. Better shielding of pulse generators has provided improvement in these areas.

10. Other sources of electromagnetic interference include: radar, microwave ovens, electric ranges, alternating magnetic fields, television transmission, and muscular activity. This list will probably grow as future scientific developments come into practical use.

11. Weapons detectors may cause a mild effect on atrioventricular (A-V) sequential and A-V synchronous pacemakers because of the low sensing threshold (0.5 mV) and unipolar design of these instruments. By and large, however, airport weapons detectors are safe for individuals with artificial pacemakers.

12. Some domestic appliances may cause a minimal effect, e.g., the loss of a beat in certain models.

13. Radiation therapy per se does not appreciably affect demand pacemaker function, but other sources of electromagnetic interference may exist in radiation therapy suites that have some effect.

PROTECTION FROM ELECTROMAGNETIC INTERFERENCE

What can the physician do to minimize the risk from electromagnetic interferences to the patient?

1. Pulse generators can have better shielding and circuitry. Pacemaker manufacturers have already made significant improvements in these areas and will no doubt continue to improve their product.

2. The physician can urge that all hospital and office equipment be well grounded and meet rigid safety specifications.

3. Most important, the physician can inform the patient with an artificial pacemaker of the potential hazards so that both physician and patient may remain vigilant concerning new exposures to possible electromagnetic interference. When these are known to exist, a safe trial must be arranged, preferably with a physician present, in which the artificial pacemaker is exposed while the patient is monitored. If there is any doubt about the resistance of a particular pacemaker to electromagnetic interference, the manufacturer should be consulted. Using these precautions, environmental hazards to the pacemaker patient may be kept to a minimum.

Artificial Pacing and Digitalis Toxicity

10

It is extremely important to remember that any patient with an artificial pacemaker (any type) by no means is immune to digitalis intoxication (DI). However, the electrocardiographic (ECG) manifestations of digitalis toxicity may be somewhat different when the cardiac rhythm is controlled by an artificial pacemaker. Except for digitalis-induced atrioventricular (A-V) block (any degree), which cannot manifest in the presence of an artificial pacemaker-induced ventricular rhythm, every known type of digitalis-induced cardiac arrhythmia can be recognized by careful examination of the ECG in patients with artificial pacemakers.

The most important clue to the diagnosis of DI is the recognition of an altered atrial mechanism, particularly the appearance of regularly occurring independent retrograde P waves in the presence of artificial pacemaker-induced ventricular rhythm. The next important diagnostic clue is to recognize frequent ventricular premature contractions (VPCs). It should be noted that there are many patients who require long-term digitalization after artificial pacing. Hence it is not unusual to see DI in patients with artificial pacemakers, although the problem often goes unrecognized. Digitalis-induced cardiac arrhythmias after artificial pacing are summarized in Table 10-1. Representative ECG manifestations of digitalis toxicity after artificial pacing are illustrated in this chapter.

Nonparoxysmal A-V Junctional Tachycardia in the Presence of Pacemaker Rhythm

1. It has been well documented that nonparoxysmal A-V junctional tachycardia is the most common digitalis-induced cardiac arrhythmia. This is also true in patients with artificial pacemakers.

2. The diagnosis of nonparoxysmal A-V junctional tachycardia is established by recognizing regularly occurring independent retrograde P waves in the presence of pacemaker rhythm (Figure 10-1).

TABLE 10-1. Digitalis-Induced Cardiac Arrhythmias after Artificial Pacing

1. Alteration of atrial activity
   a. Nonparoxysmal A-V junctional tachycardia with pacemaker rhythm
   b. Atrial tachycardia with pacemaker rhythm
   c. A-V junctional escape rhythm with pacemaker rhythm
   d. Sinus bradycardia with pacemaker rhythm
   e. Sinus arrest or sinoatrial block with pacemaker rhythm
2. Ventricular arrhythmias
   a. Ventricular premature contractions with pacemaker rhythm
   b. Ventricular tachycardia or fibrillation
3. Rare digitalis-induced arrhythmias
   a. Reciprocal beats or rhythm with pacemaker rhythm
   b. Atrial fibrillation of flutter with pacemaker rhythm

3. The usual rate in nonparoxysmal A-V junctional tachycardia ranges from 70 to 130 beats/min.

4. Nonparoxysmal A-V junctional tachycardia is frequently unrecognized in this circumstance simply because many physicians do not pay attention to the atrial mechanism after artificial pacing.

5. Nonparoxysmal A-V junctional focus activates the entire heart from time to time, so that the artificial pacemaker-induced ventricular beats occur only intermittently in the presence of underlying nonparoxysmal A-V junctional tachycardia.

6. Other digitalis-induced cardiac arrhythmias, particularly VPCs may coexist.

The alteration in the atrial mechanism is the most important finding for diagnosing digitalis toxicity in patients with artificial pacemakers.

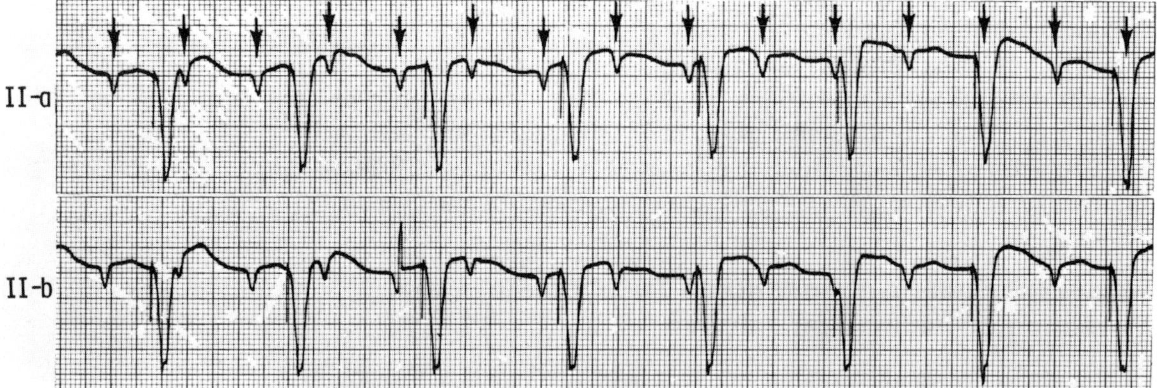

FIGURE 10-1. Leads II-a and II-b are not continuous. *Arrows* indicate retrograde P waves. The rhythm is nonparoxysmal A-V junctional tachycardia (atrial rate: 100 beats/min) in the presence of artificial pacemaker-induced ventricular rhythm. DI is the underlying cause of the A-V junctional tachycardia.

VPCs in the Presence of Pacemaker Rhythm

1. The frequent occurrence of VPCs is readily recognized in DI, even in patients with artificial pacemakers, because the cardiac rhythm change in this case is obvious to most physicians (Figure 10-2).

2. When the fixed-rate ventricular pacemaker is used, VPCs are commonly interpolated.

3. On the other hand, the artificial pacemaker cycle is reset by the VPCs when the demand pacemaker is used.

4. One of the important findings in patients with artificial pacemakers is that there may be significant pulse deficits resulting from insufficient cardiac output by the VPCs. This is induced by digitalis because of mechanicoelectrical dissociation (Figure 10-2). Thus many elderly individuals with advanced heart disease develop significant symptoms, e.g., hypotension, dizziness, aggravation of congestive heart failure (CHF), or even fainting, in this circumstance.

5. Digitalis-induced VPCs may coexist with other arrhythmias, e.g., nonparoxysmal A-V junctional tachycardia.

6. In far advanced cases of DI, VPCs may lead to ventricular tachycardia or fibrillation and even death in spite of the artificial pacing.

Sinus Bradyarrhythmias in the Presence of Pacemaker Rhythm

1. When the patient develops digitalis toxicity after a permanent pacemaker implantation, various sinus bradyarrhythmias may be observed in the presence of pacemaker rhythm.

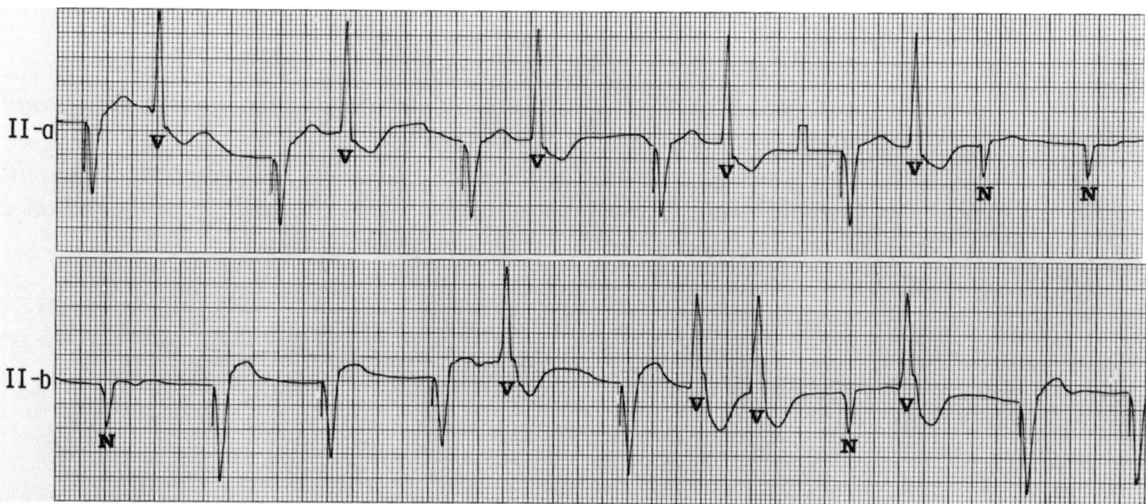

FIGURE 10-2. Leads II-a and II-b are continuous. The basic rhythm is AF with a demand ventricular pacemaker-induced rhythm and intermittent nonparoxysmal A-V junctional tachycardia (*N*) with frequent VPCs (*V*). Note that the interval from the patient's own beat to the pacemaker beat is longer than the consecutively occurring pacemaker interval because of hysteresis.

2. The most common digitalis-induced sinus bradyarrhythmia is sinus bradycardia.

3. Less commonly, sinus arrest or sinoatrial block (either Mobitz type I or II) may be observed.

4. In this circumstance, of course, the sinus P waves are not conducted to the ventricles because of the underlying complete A-V block in many cases.

A-V Junctional Escape Rhythm in the Presence of Pacemaker Rhythm

1. Less commonly, A-V junctional escape rhythm may develop because of digitalis toxicity in the presence of pacemaker rhythm.

2. Electrocardiographically, A-V junctional escape rhythm is diagnosed in the presence of pacemaker-induced ventricular rhythm by recognizing independent, regularly occurring retrograde P waves with a slow rate (40 to 60 beats/min).

3. In other words, A-V junctional pacemaker activates the atria in a retrograde fashion while the artificial pacemaker controls the ventricular activity independently in this circumstance.

Atrial Tachycardia in the Presence of Pacemaker Rhythm

1. Although atrial tachycardia associated with varying degrees of A-V block [paroxysmal atrial tachycardia (PAT) with block, most commonly Wenckebach A-V block] is considered to be almost pathognomonic for digitalis toxicity, its occurrence is not very common compared with the presence of nonparoxysmal A-V junctional tachycardia or VPCs in DI.

2. For the same reason, digitalis-induced atrial tachycardia in the presence of artificial pacemaker-induced ventricular rhythm is not very common.

3. On the ECG, independent and rapid (160 to 250 beats/min) upright P waves (lead II) are observed in this circumstance in the presence of artificial pacemaker-induced ventricular rhythm.

Artificial Pacing: Complications and Malfunctions

11

Although biomedical as well as engineering aspects of artificial cardiac pacing have improved enormously during the past decade, various complications and malfunctions (Table 11-1) are still associated with artificial pacemakers. Fortunately, however, serious manifestations of malfunctioning pacemakers, e.g., runaway pacemaker, are relatively uncommon at the present time because of the ready availability of reliable pacemaker follow-up care, including artificial pacemaker clinics and transtelephone pacemaker monitoring systems (see Chapters 1 and 12). Hence, far-advanced malfunctions of artificial pacing can be easily avoided. In addition, the general knowledge of most practicing physicians regarding artificial pacing has been improved significantly in recent years so that various complications, e.g., infections, perforation of the heart, and malposition of the pacemaker electrode, can be minimized. Furthermore, valuable information regarding the interrelationship between various drugs (e.g., procainamide), electrolyte imbalance (e.g., hyper- or hypokalemia), and artificial pacemakers is available to clinicians, and certain avoidable pacemaker malfunctions may be prevented (see Chapter 9). Clinical data regarding various electromagnetic sources which may interfere with the artificial pacemaker functions have also been accumulating, and this information is invaluable in terms of learning to avoid certain pacemaker malfunctions (see Chapter 9).

During the insertion or implantation of an artificial pacemaker, the danger of inducing ventricular fibrillation (VF) is always possible, and therefore a defibrillator must be immediately available. Various commonly used cardiac emergency drugs, including all of the antiarrhythmic agents, should be on hand as well. Some cardiac arrhythmias (e.g., VF) caused by malfunctioning pacemakers are so serious that sudden death may occur. On the other hand, some cardiac rhythm changes are related to the artificial pacemaker and are *not* due to a true malfunction. The term pseudomalfunction may be used in this circumstance. Otherwise,

TABLE 11-1. Complications and Malfunctions of Artificial Cardiac Pacing

1. Malfunctioning pacemakers
   a. Acceleration of pacing (runaway pacemaker)
   b. Slowing of pacing
   c. Irregular pacing
   d. Failure of sensing
   e. Failure of capture
   f. Any combination of the above
2. Ventricular fibrillation
3. Perforation of the heart
4. Infections
5. Thromboembolic phenomena
6. Pacemaker sounds
7. Miscellaneous
   a. Electrode fracture
   b. Knotting of wire
   c. Inhibition of pacemaker by noncardiac muscle potentials
   d. Hypotension and cardiac failure
   e. Bowel necrosis
   f. Displacement of pulse generator
   g. Electromagnetic interference
   h. Electrocardiographic interference
   i. Social and psychological problems

certain cardiac rhythm disturbances simply coexist with the pacemaker rhythm and are totally unrelated to the artificial pacemaker. It is extremely important to distinguish between a true malfunction and pseudomalfunction of the artificial pacemaker.

DIAGNOSTIC APPROACH

Distinguishing true malfunctions of the electronic and mechanical factors from physiological problems or pseudomalfunctions which are related to artificial pacing or which coexist with normally functioning pacemaker rhythm is essential. Proper management and other therapeutic approaches can be established only by correctly diagnosing the various problems and complications associated with artificial pacing. The diagnostic approach may include careful history taking, physical examination, electrocardiographic (ECG) analysis, x-ray examination, and specific electronic analysis of pacemaker function.

History Taking

The simplest and yet most important diagnostic approach is careful history taking.

1. The patient should be asked if any symptoms, particularly dizziness, near-syncope, or syncope, similar or identical to those which he experienced before pacing have recurred after artificial pacemaker implantation. The recurrence of such symptoms may indicate pacemaker malfunction, especially failure of cardiac capture.

2. The "pacemaker syndrome" may be suspected when the patient develops rhythmic waves of weakness suggestive of orthostatic hypotension.

3. When there are other complaints, e.g., palpitations, skipped heart beats, or irregular heart beats, the patient is most likely experiencing extrasystoles—commonly ventricular premature contractions (VPCs) and, less commonly, atrial or atrioventricular (A-V) junctional premature contractions—or an intermittent appearance of the patient's own natural beats (sinus or ectopic). The premature beats may be spontaneous or induced by the artificial pacemaker.

4. On the other hand, palpitations may be caused by the loss of consecutive sensing and/or capture, or competition between the patient's natural rhythm and the fixed-rate pacemaker-induced ventricular rhythm.

5. When the patient complains of near-syncope or syncope after artificial pacing, the problem may indicate intermittent capture after lead fracture, reduction of the pacing output, increased threshold beyond the output capability of the pulse generator, electrode displacement, or even perforation of the ventricles.

6. When the patient develops hypotension and/or congestive heart failure (CHF) after artificial pacing, the finding suggests that cardiac output and peripheral arterial pressure are reduced because of a lack of atrial contribution during ventricular pacing. Another type of pacing, e.g., atrial-synchronized or bifocal pacing, is recommended under this circumstance (see Chapter 1).

7. When any new symptoms (e.g., chest pain) are observed, of course, an appropriate diagnostic approach (e.g., serum enzyme study, cardiac nuclear imaging, ECG) is in order.

8. In a case of significant CHF, the patient may be digitalized with or without diuretic therapy.

9. It is important to reemphasize that no one is immune to any cardiac disease [e.g., acute myocardial infarction (MI), CHF, or pulmonary embolism] or drug toxicity, particularly digitalis intoxication (DI), even after artificial pacing (see Chapter 10).

Physical Examination

Needless to say, it is essential to perform a complete physical examination during follow-up visits on each patient with a permanent artificial pacemaker.

1. The physician should pay particular attention to any new complaint.

2. During inspection, the gross appearance of the surgical wound (e.g., the presence or absence of infection), the location of the pulse generator (e.g., normal versus abnormal location), the presence or absence of any obvious distress (e.g., dyspnea, pain), and any other striking findings can be easily evaluated.

3. Although some discomfort may be expected around the surgical wound for a few weeks after pacemaker implantation, persistent local

pain is definitely an abnormal finding. When this is present, the physician should check to see if the pacemaker skin pocket is too tight or if the pulse generator is displaced to an undesired location.

4. More importantly, the presence or absence of infection should be carefully determined. The surgical wound may be infected with a rapidly growing organism (e.g., *Staphylococcus aureus*) or a slowly growing organism (e.g., *Staphylococcus epidermidis*).

5. In the absence of infection, local pain or discomfort may be caused by a wound decubitus or pressure necrosis of the skin, with the skin actually being broken down.

6. In addition, the pacemaker may be in a skin fold, causing marked discomfort.

7. Furthermore, the local pain or profound discomfort may be induced by the pulse generator rubbing against the arm with each movement when the apparatus is located in the axilla or in the anterior axillary fold. These local problems should be eliminated promptly (see Management).

8. When the patient complains of chest pain suggestive of angina or chest discomfort of a similar nature, the diagnosis of true angina pectoris or even acute MI should be suspected.

9. Vital signs provide invaluable information regarding the patient's well-being as well as about the status of the artificial cardiac pacing.

10. For example, hypotension or evidence of CHF may indicate an improper mode of pacing. That is, the patient may require atrial-synchronized pacing or bifocal pacing by utilizing atrial contribution to enhance the cardiac output when the ventricular pacing is not sufficient to maintain minimum cardiac output. Alternatively, the patient may require digitalization in addition to artificial pacing.

11. A pulse rate that is significantly slower or faster than the preset pacing rate is strongly indicative of pacemaker malfunction.

12. Infection is obviously suspected when the patient is febrile.

13. The nature of the cardiac rhythm—whether too slow, too fast, or irregular—can be readily evaluated by careful auscultation. The auscultatory finding is later confirmed by ECG analysis (discussed later) regarding malfunctions, extrasystoles, or other abnormalities.

14. In addition to the cardiac rhythm evaluation, abnormal sounds or friction rubs related to the artificial pacemaker can be appreciated (discussed later).

15. The presence or absence of thromboembolic phenomena, particularly pulmonary embolism or infarction, should be carefully evaluated when any clinical suspicion is raised (discussed later).

Laboratory Tests

Various laboratory tests, particularly the 12-lead ECG, ECG rhythm strips (commonly leads II and V_1), the Holter monitor ECG, and chest x-rays, are frequently used to assess pacemaker function in addition to the usual history taking and physical examination. In many medical centers more sophisticated electronic analysis of the artificial pacemaker function can be performed.

Electrocardiogram

1. Any long ECG rhythm strip (commonly leads II, V_1, or V_6) which show the pacemaker artifact most clearly should be used for the cardiac rhythm analysis.

2. The ECG can identify various malfunctions of artificial pacemakers, including acceleration of pacing (runaway pacemaker), slowing of pacing, irregular pacing, failure of sensing and/or capture, and any combinations of the above (Table 11-1).

3. In addition, various cardiac arrhythmias which coexist with the pacemaker rhythm (not caused by a malfunction) can be detected.

4. The ECG may indicate the lead disruption by recognizing the alteration of the vector in the artificial pacemaker artifacts. Lead disruption is strongly indicated when intermittent failure of stimulation occurs, especially in conjunction with intermittent reduction of the amplitude in the stimulus artifact.

5. Acute MI, perforation of the ventricles (discussed later), and various other acute cardiac events may be diagnosed from the 12-lead ECG.

Holter Monitor ECG

When pacemaker malfunction is strongly suspected but the conventional ECG (including long rhythm strips) fails to confirm the diagnosis, the Holter monitor ECG should be performed. Any intermittent nature of pacemaker malfunction, e.g., intermittent failure of cardiac capture, can be readily documented by the Holter monitor ECG.

X-ray Examination

The x-ray examination can provide confirmation of displacement of the lead within the heart, lifting of the infected myocardial electrodes from the surface of the heart, and a fractured intramyocardial lead. The radiological analysis of the pulse generator itself can provide useful information as to the status of the energy source.

Electronic Analysis

1. When artificial pacemaker malfunction is not documented by the history taking, physical examination, 12-lead ECG, x-ray examination, and Holter monitor ECG, the patient should be connected to the ECG and oscilloscope for electronic analysis of the generator artifact.

2. The sensitive indicator of the integrity of the lead-connector system is the display of the pulse generator stimulus on the oscilloscope. The normal output of the pulse generator in a normally functioning pacing system versus a failure of sensing and/or capture caused by lead disruption can be clearly distinguished by display of the artifact at a rapid sweep and with proper equipment.

3. Certain provocative maneuvers with electronic analysis of the pacemaker function are necessary in some situations. The pulse generator and electrode should be manipulated in the subcutaneous tissue by changing the patient's body position in various ways (e.g., turning side to side, lying, standing, bending, straightening). These maneuvers may demonstrate a partially disrupted lead or connector that is producing the failure of sensing and/or capture by displaying the change on the oscilloscope.

Follow-up Care

It is essential to provide proper follow-up care for all patients with permanent artificial pacemakers in order to detect early malfunction and prevent major complications of artificial pacing (see Chapters 1 and 12).

MANIFESTATIONS OF COMPLICATIONS AND MALFUNCTIONS OF ARTIFICIAL PACING

The complications and malfunctions of artificial pacing are summarized in Table 11-1. It is extremely important to distinguish between the true malfunctions and the pseudomalfunctions.

Malfunctioning Pacemakers

A malfunctioning pacemaker may manifest its problem by alterations of the preset pacing rate (acceleration or slowing), irregular pacing, failure of sensing, failure of cardiac capture, or any combination of the above (Table 11-1).

Acceleration of Pacing (Runaway Pacemaker)

1. A malfunctioning pacemaker should be suspected even if the pacing rate is accelerated only one or two beats compared with the preset rate, providing the equipment used to measure the heart rate is in perfect condition.

2. The term runaway pacemaker is used when the artificial pacing rate is accelerated so that pacemaker-induced ventricular tachycardia (VT) is produced (Figure 11-1).

3. Until 10 to 15 years ago, when the fixed-rate pacemaker started to be used less frequently, runaway pacemaker was a common manifestation of the malfunctioning pacemaker.

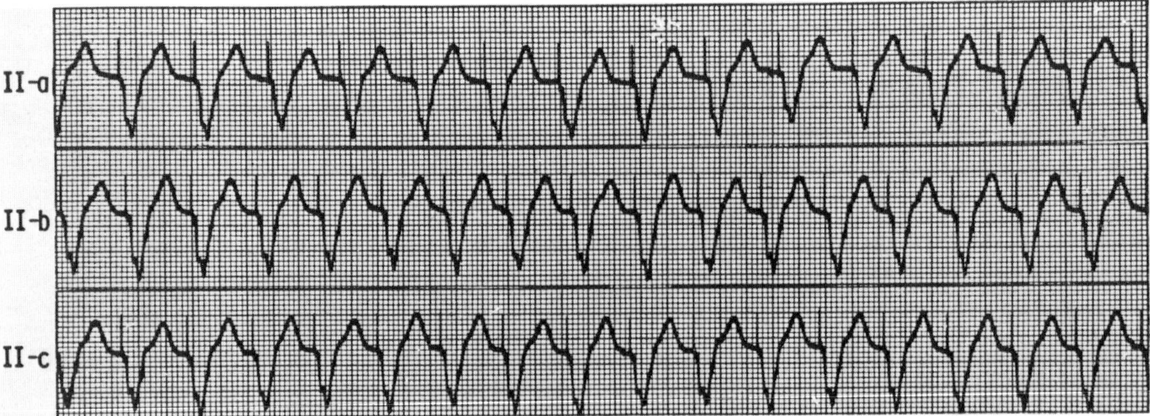

FIGURE 11-1. Leads II-a, II-b, and II-c are not continuous. The tracing shows an artificial pacemaker-induced ventricular tachycardia (rate: 105 to 125 beats/min)—runaway pacemaker. Note that the preset pacing rate in this patient was 70 beats/min.

4. Fortunately, the runaway pacemaker has been encountered much less commonly since the demand ventricular pacemaker has been gradually replacing the fixed-rate model, particularly in the United States.

5. Nevertheless, runaway pacemaker may be observed with almost all types of artificial pacemaker (including old and new models) regardless of manufacturer.

6. When the pacing rate of the runaway pacemaker is exceedingly enhanced, the preexisting bradyarrhythmias (often high degree or complete A-V block) reappear because failure of sensing and cardiac capture usually occur together (Figure 11-2).

7. The usual pacing rate of the runaway pacemaker ranges from 80 to 160 beats/min (Figure 11-1), but the pacing rate may be increased to as fast as 450 to 1,000 beats/min (Figure 11-2).

8. Runaway pacemaker may be associated with irregular pacing.

9. VF may occur in far-advanced runaway pacemaker and may lead to sudden death.

10. On the other hand, VF also can occur even in the patient with a normally functioning pacemaker (Figure 11-3).

11. Antitachyarrhythmic agents, needless to say, are ineffective for runaway pacemaker. Runaway pacemaker is a medical emergency which should be treated immediately (discussed under Management).

Slowing of Pacing

Slowing of the pacing rate is a more common manifestation of malfunction when the demand mode is used. The slowing of the pacing may have a regular rhythm (Figure 11-4), although it may also be associated with irregular pacing (Figure 11-5). Extremely slow pacing often produces a syncopal attack as a result of a long ventricular standstill (Figure 11-5). In an advanced case of malfunction, the pacing rate may be grossly irregular.

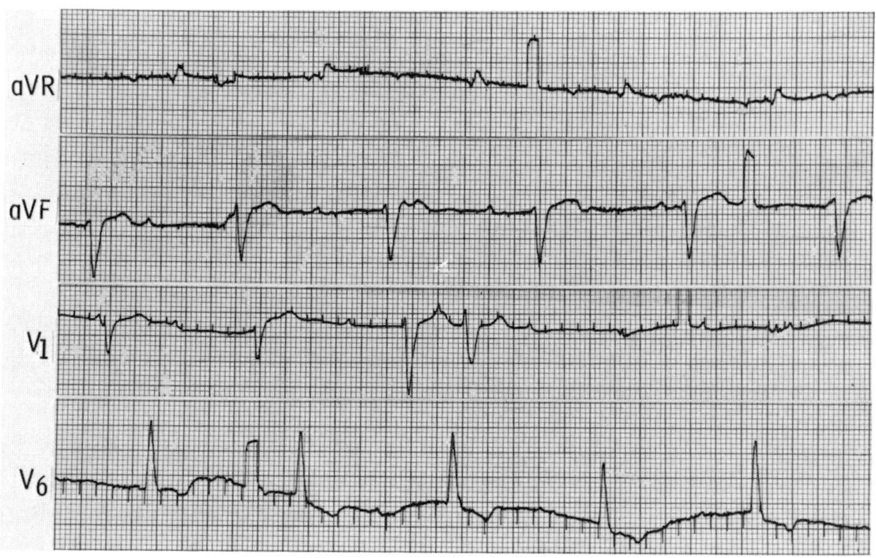

FIGURE 11-2. The pacing rate is extremely rapid (480 beats/min) so that none of the pacing impulses are followed by the QRS complex. As a result, a preexisting complete A-V block has reappeared. This ECG tracing is an example of a far-advanced runaway pacemaker. Note the VPC in lead V_1.

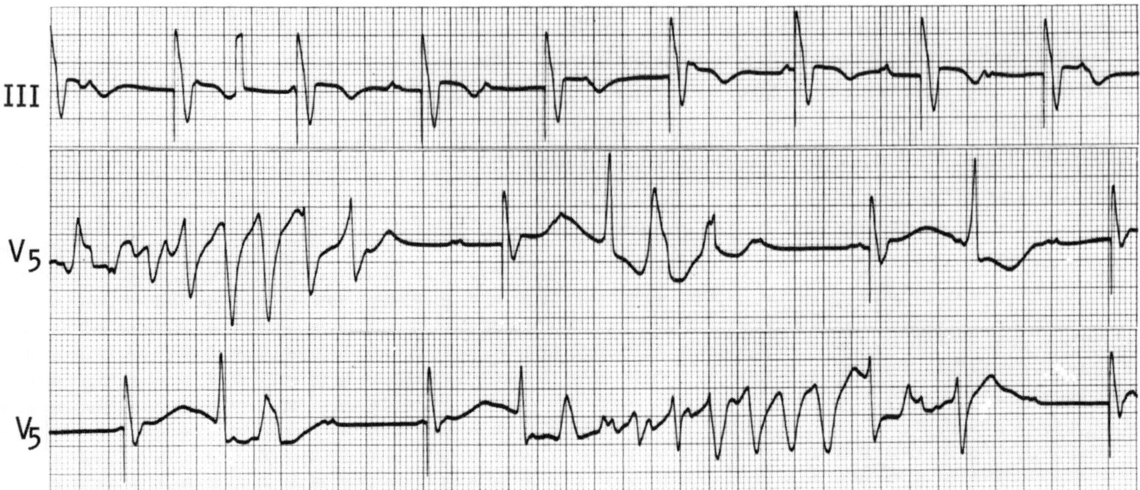

FIGURE 11-3. Artificial pacemaker (demand unit) induced ventricular rhythm with paroxysmal ventricular fibrillation because of the R-on-T phenomenon. The atrial mechanism is sinus. The R-R interval from the patient's natural beat to the next pacemaker beat is longer than the present pacing interval because of hysteresis. The pacemaker functions normally.

Irregular Pacing

An irregular pacing rate usually indicates an advanced form of malfunction. The irregular pacing may be associated with acceleration or slowing of the pacing rate (Figure 11-5).

Failure of Sensing

Failure of sensing may occur as an isolated finding, although it is commonly associated with a failure of cardiac capture. It is common expe-

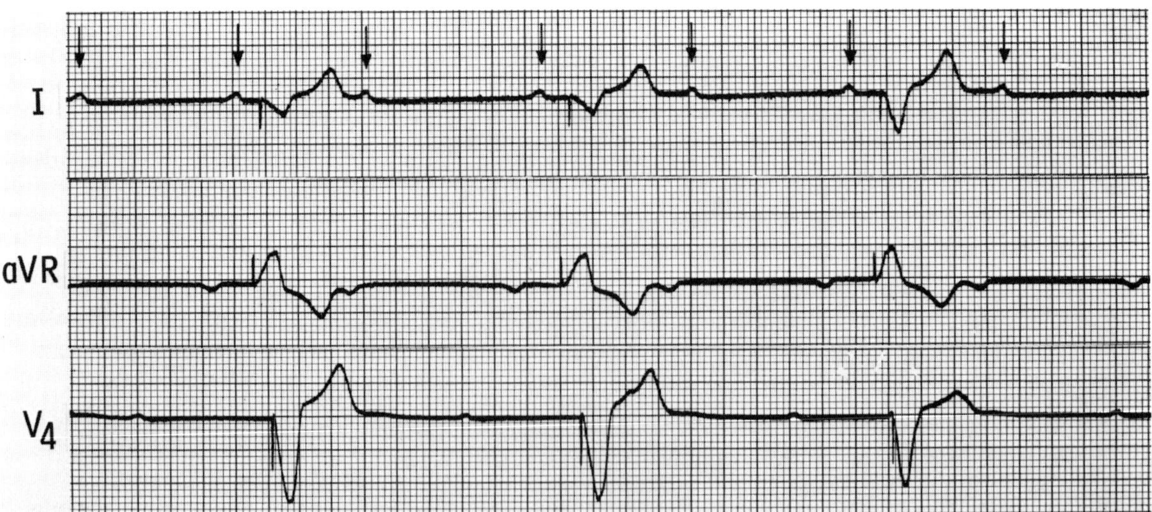

FIGURE 11-4. The *arrows* indicate sinus P waves. A malfunctioning demand pacemaker is manifested by the extremely slow pacing rate of 31 beats/min. The preset pacing rate of this patient was 70 beats/min.

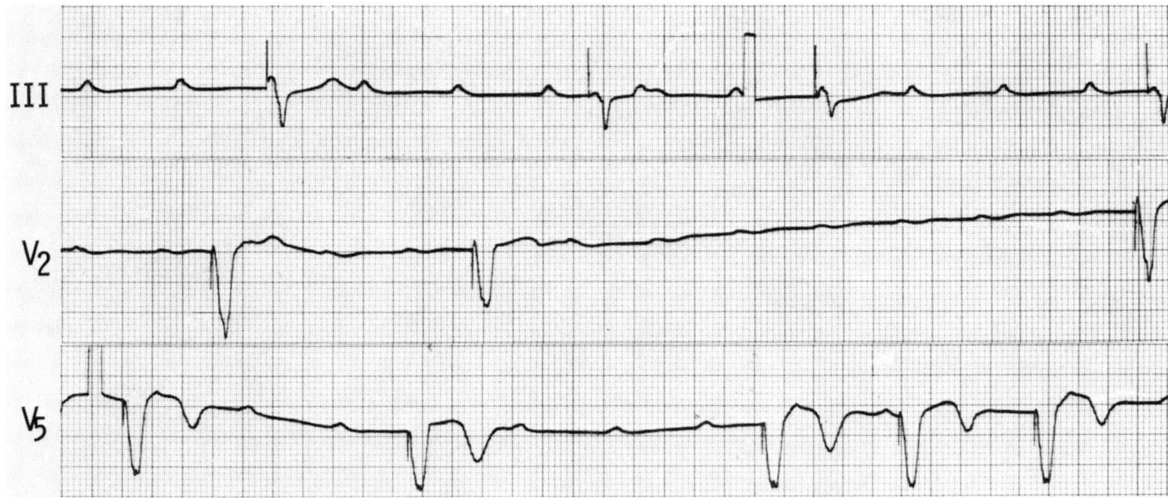

FIGURE 11-5. Malfunctioning pacemaker is manifested by a markedly slow and irregular pacing rhythm.

rience that a demand unit functions as a fixed mode when a sensing device does not work properly.

Failure of Cardiac Capture

1. Failure of cardiac capture may be complete, but it is nearly always intermittent (Figure 11-6).

2. At times improper capture of the ventricles by the artificial pacemaker is manifested by Wenckebach exit block of the pacing impulses.

3. The patient may develop a near-syncope or even a true syncope when a long ventricular standstill is produced by consecutive failure of the cardiac capture.

4. During failure of cardiac capture by the artificial pacemaker, the preexisting bradyarrhythmias (commonly complete A-V block) may reappear. Otherwise, a long ventricular standstill is often observed with consecutive nonconducted sinus P waves resulting from failure of ventricular capture.

5. The most common cause of failure of cardiac capture is probably malposition of the pacemaker electrode and electrode fracture. Catheter displacement is reported to occur in 6 to 45% of all permanent transvenous catheter implantations. The catheter displacement may be observed at any time, but it often occurs within the first month after implantation.

6. Otherwise, failure of cardiac capture may be caused by fibrosis around the pacemaker electrode, advancement of the underlying heart disease, severe hyper- or hypokalemia, or drug toxicity, e.g., quinidine or procainamide (see Chapter 9).

7. When the above-mentioned factors are not present, the pacemaker itself is probably malfunctioning. Runaway pacemaker with an extremely rapid pacing rate is nearly always associated with failure of ventricular capture (Figure 11-2).

Any Combination of the Above

Combinations of the above-mentioned manifestations often exist, especially with advanced malfunctioning pacemakers. For example, as men-

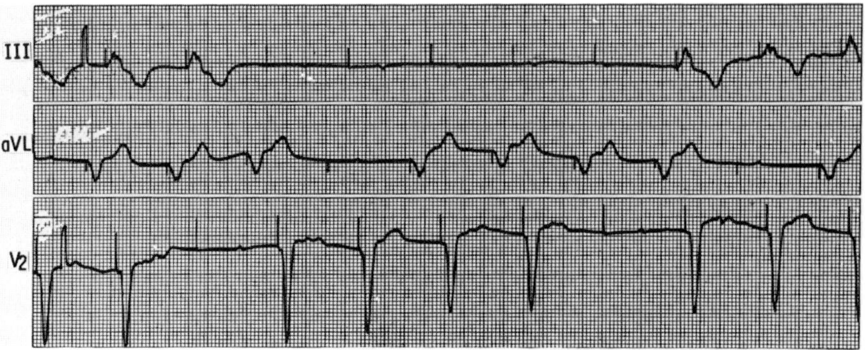

FIGURE 11-6. Artificial pacemaker-induced ventricular rhythm with frequent failure of ventricular capture resulting in areas of ventricular standstill.

tioned previously, runaway pacemaker with a very rapid pacing rate (more than 300 beats/min) is almost always associated with failure of sensing as well as failure of cardiac capture (Figure 11-2). Another example is irregular pacing, which is usually associated with acceleration or slowing of the pacing rate (Figure 11-5).

Ventricular Fibrillation

1. Ventricular fibrillation (VF) may occur in any patient during insertion or implantation of the artificial pacemaker, especially when the threshold of the VF is expected to be low, e.g., in acute MI.

2. It is also a known fact that VF is frequently produced when the pacemaker artifact is superimposed during the vulnerable period of the ventricles as a result of the R-on-T phenomenon (Figure 11-7).

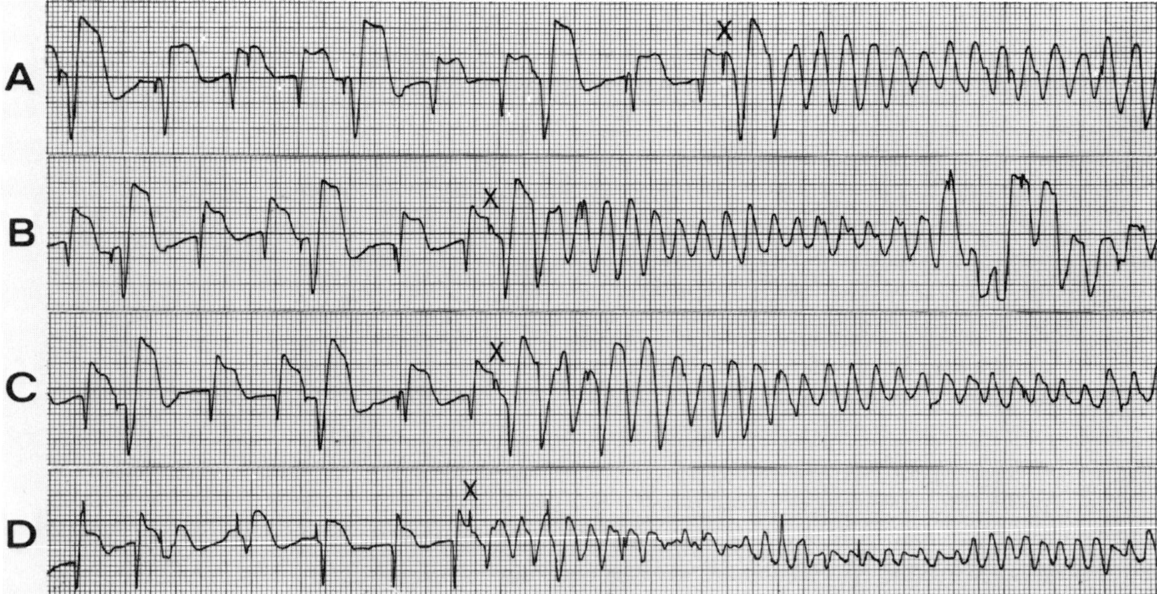

FIGURE 11-7. Rhythm strips **A** to **D** represent a monitor lead; they are not continuous. Ventricular fibrillation is initiated by the artificial pacemaker (fixed-rate) spike (*X*) because of the R-on-T phenomenon.

3. On the other hand, VF may be produced as a result of far-advanced runaway pacemaker.

4. It should be noted that VF may occur and be entirely unrelated to the artificial pacemaker (Figure 11-3).

5. VF may also be associated with infectious complications after pacing.

Perforation of the Heart

Perforation of the heart, especially the ventricles, can occur, particularly when a transvenous catheter electrode is used. Perforation of the ventricles may be suspected when the following findings occur:

1. *Right bundle branch block (RBBB) pattern.* Although RBBB pattern of the paced beats strongly suggests perforation of the ventricles, particularly the ventricular septum, it may be observed in coronary sinus pacing beats and even on normal right ventricular paced beats in the absence of perforation.

2. *Intercostal muscle or diaphragmatic contraction.* Myocardial perforation is suggested when intercostal muscle or diaphragmatic contraction occurs as a result of pacing stimuli. Usually diaphragmatic and intercostal pacing occurs in patients whose pacemaker electrode is in the right ventricular cavity.

3. *Pericarditis, pericardial effusion, or cardiac tamponade.* Pericardial friction rub often suggests myocardial perforation, but cardiac tamponade is a very rare complication. It should be noted, however, that a friction rub is frequently observed in patients with a normal endocardial electrode position without myocardial perforation.

4. *Heart murmur or friction rubs.* Pansystolic murmur may result from rupture of the ventricular septum. In addition, various cardiac valves, particularly the tricuspid valve, may be damaged or lacerated by the pacemaker electrode, leading to various heart murmurs. Furthermore, friction rub may be caused by myocardial perforation by the transvenous pacemaker electrodes (see also Pacemaker Sounds).

In addition to the characteristic ECG and auscultatory findings, in most cases perforation of the heart can be diagnosed by x-ray examination, which demonstrates the malpositioned catheter electrode.

Infections

1. Infectious complications of transvenous pacemaker implantation have been reported in approximately 5 to 6% of patients. The infections commonly involve the pacemaker generator pocket.

2. The mortality rate from the infectious complications has been estimated to be about 2%.

3. The most common infecting organisms are *Staphylococcus aureus* and *Staph. albus*.

4. Sustained bacteremia or endocarditis is still a relatively uncom-

mon complication. However, if it occurs, a serious therapeutic dilemma is frequently encountered.

5. Eradication of infection is extremely difficult unless the pacemaker generator or the catheter electrode is removed. Furthermore, removal of the pacemaker electrode may require major intracardiac surgery because with the passage of time the electrode is often firmly fixed to the endocardial surface.

6. Nonetheless, endocarditis has reported to be apparently cured using combined antibiotic therapy without removal of the pacemaker electrode.

7. Sepsis involving the pacemaker generator usually develops shortly after implantation (median time: 2.5 weeks), whereas electrode catheter infection often occurs later (median time: 33 weeks), after erosion of the electrode loop in the neck. The risk of generator sepsis usually increases with each subsequent replacement.

Thromboembolic Phenomena

1. Thromboembolic complications after implantation of permanent pacemakers are rare, but if they occur the outcome is often fatal.

2. Pulmonary embolism and infarction are the most common causes of death in these circumstances.

3. Pulmonary embolism may result from thrombosis around the pacemaker electrode in the superior vena cava, the right atrium, or the right ventricle.

4. A large right atrial thrombus surrounding the permanent transvenous pacemaker catheter has been reported.

5. Axillary-subclavian vein thrombosis along the course of the catheter and cerebral dural venous sinus thrombosis after cardiac pacemaker implantation have also been reported.

6. Thromboembolic phenomena should be suspected in all patients with permanent pacemakers when they develop unexplained dyspnea, tachycardia, chest pain, or refractory heart failure. Early recognition with proper management (e.g., anticoagulant therapy) of the thromboembolic phenomena may prevent major complications and even death.

Pacemaker Sounds

A variety of interesting auscultatory findings can be observed after artificial cardiac pacing. The term pacemaker sounds has been used to describe various extra heart sounds related to the artificial pacing. The nature of these pacemaker sounds depends on the mode of artificial pacing, the position of the pacing electrode, the atrial mechanism, and the status of A-V and intraventricular conduction. In many cases, malposition of the pacemaker electrode has been the cause of the sounds. On the other hand, some investigators think that the pacemaker sound is often of academic interest only, and therefore repositioning the catheter tip is not indicated. When friction rubs are present, however, silent myocardial perforation may be suspected, and extensive diagnostic procedures and even repositioning of the pacemaker electrode may be necessary.

Pacemaker Click

1. The most frequent auscultatory finding after pacing is probably a high frequency presystolic click which occurs approximately 6 msec after the pacing spike.

2. Initially, the pacemaker click was thought to be of cardiac origin, but recent experience indicates that it is related to intercostal or diaphragmatic stimulation by the pacing electrode.

3. By and large, the pacemaker click is considered to be a benign, clinically insignificant auscultatory finding.

4. Nevertheless, the pacemaker click has been noted in some cases with silent myocardial perforation or partial penetration of the electrode into the right ventricular myocardium.

Heart Murmurs

1. Pansystolic or late systolic murmurs have been reported after pacing. The quality of the murmurs is described as a superficial scratch sound in some cases.

2. The systolic murmur is often attributed to tricuspid insufficiency induced by the pacing catheter.

3. Laceration of the tricuspid valve and fibrinous adhesion of the pacemaker catheter to the tricuspid valve have been observed in some cases, but most of these lesions have been documented at postmortem examination and were not suspected clinically.

4. Another sound, described as "cardiac whoop," was reported in a patient with MI after temporary transvenous pacing. Movement of the pacing wire in the right ventricular cavity was thought to be the origin of the sound. The cardiac whoop is clinically insignificant.

Friction Rubs

1. In the past, myocardial perforation was strongly suspected in every case in which the patient with an artificial pacemaker developed a friction rub in the absence of acute MI or in any other clinical setting that would cause acute pericarditis.

2. However, there are several documented reports indicating that a friction rub may occur in paced patients with no evidence of myocardial perforation.

3. It has been suggested that the friction rub in this circumstance is due to contact of the pacing wire with the inner surface of the myocardium. Thus the term endocardial friction rub has been used.

4. As seen with the usual pericardial friction rub, the endocardial friction rub may also be audible during the three phases of the cardiac cycle when the ventricles move rapidly: with early rapid diastolic filling of the ventricles, in response to accelerated ventricular filling after atrial contraction, and with ventricular systole.

5. As expected, the endocardial friction rub usually disappears as soon as the pacing catheter is withdrawn from the right ventricle to the right atrium.

Miscellaneous Problems

In addition to the above findings, many other problems can be encountered in patients with artificial pacemakers.

Electrode Fracture

Electrode fracture usually manifests as a failure of sensing and/or cardiac capture, as discussed previously.

Knotting of the Wire

On rare occasions, knotting of the wire occurs when a markedly flexible pacing wire is utilized. Extreme care should be taken whenever the highly flexible temporary pacing wire is in the ventricle while a permanent pacing electrode catheter is being introduced.

Inhibition of Pacemaker by Noncardiac Muscle Potentials

1. Inhibition of demand pacemakers by musculoskeletal potentials is relatively common when unipolar pacing systems are utilized.

2. Inhibition of bipolar demand pacemakers by noncardiac muscle potentials, however, is a relatively uncommon phenomenon which has been reported only recently. Bipolar demand modes are not prone to noncardiac muscle potential inhibition because the relative proximity of the pacing electrodes causes a lower potential difference between the poles.

3. Inhibition of demand pacing is often caused by the pectoralis major muscle potentials, but it may be due to myopotentials originating from the anterior abdominal wall muscles or diaphragmatic myopotentials.

4. Thus transient pacemaker inhibition may be induced by active contraction of the diaphragm, e.g., deep inspiration, straining, Valsalva maneuver, coughing, sneezing, and laughing.

5. Demand pacemaker inhibition may be prevented by the wider use of bipolar pacing electrodes. Otherwise, fixed-rate pacing can eliminate this type of interference.

Hypotension and Cardiac Failure

When the atrial contribution is essential to maintain adequate cardiac output for daily activity, the asynchronous (ventricular) pacemaker provides no beneficial effect. In fact, hypotension and cardiac failure may result from the reduced cardiac output during ventricular pacing because of a loss of atrial contribution to left ventricular filling. Therefore, atrial synchronized pacing or bifocal demand pacing (see Chapter 1) is definitely indicated so as to utilize the atrial contribution which can provide adequate cardiac output in these patients.

Necrosis of the Bowel

A rare instance of small bowel necrosis resulting from artificial pacemaker implantation in the abdominal wall was reported recently. It has also been suggested that placement of the artificial pacemaker in the abdominal wall between the peritoneum and the deep fascia may be hazardous. Thus it is advisable to place the pacemaker more superficially in the abdominal wall in order to avoid this rare complication.

Displacement of the Pulse Generator

Displacement of the artificial cardiac pacemaker may occur, particularly in elderly individuals with inelastic skin when a heavyweight pulse generator is used. Retraction of the endocardial electrode may be produced by the downward migration of the heavy pulse generator, and displacement of the pulse generator may, of course, produce pacing failure. This complication can be prevented by anchoring the pulse generator to the clavicle or by creating a pacemaker pocket under the pectoral major muscle.

Electromagnetic Interference

Artificial pacemaker function may be interfered with by various electromagnetic sources, including commercial radar, electric shavers, defibrillators, microwave ovens, transurethral electrocautery, small electric motors, single engine motors, a malfunctioning television set, etc. (see Chapter 9). The demand pacemaker is much more vulnerable to these electromagnetic sources than the fixed-rate pacemaker.

ECG Interference

Various electrophysiological events may cause alterations of pacemaker function. For example, the demand pacemaker may sense a tall P wave or T wave instead of the R wave. In one patient intermittent suppression of the pacemaker was caused by a prominent T wave that resulted from too close contact of the intracardiac electrode with the ventricular endocardium. In another patient, apparent malfunction of the demand pacemaker was caused by concealed ventricular extrasystoles. In addition, inhibition of a demand pacemaker by current leakage resulting from defective grounding in an ECG recorder power cable has been reported.

Social and Psychological Problems

Some anxious patients, particularly young females, are self-conscious about the cosmetic aspect of the implanted artificial pacemaker because the pulse generator with its surgical scar protrudes on the upper chest. Other patients become overly anxious about their cardiac functions after permanent pacing, and unnecessary fear of death from pacing malfunctions cannot always be avoided. These sociopsychological problems related to artificial pacemakers can often be alleviated by reassurance from the physician.

PREVENTION AND MANAGEMENT

It is important to prevent major complications related to artificial pacemakers.

Malfunctioning Pacemakers

When good follow-up care, including artificial pacemaker clinics and a transtelephone monitoring system, is provided after the implantation of permanent artificial pacemakers, major and far-advanced malfunctions can be easily prevented. Early signs of a malfunctioning pacemaker can be recognized readily and the old pacemaker replaced with a new pulse generator without delay when reliable pacemaker follow-up care is available. By doing so, serious malfunctions, e.g., runaway pacemaker, can be prevented in most cases.

1. When runaway pacemaker (Figures 11-1 and 2) is diagnosed, particularly when the patient is symptomatic (e.g., near-syncope or syncope), the malfunctioning unit should be promptly disconnected from the heart. This can be accomplished by cutting the electrode wires near their attachments to the pacemaker. Replacing a temporary pacemaker connected to the bare electrode ends usually results in the prompt recovery of most patients.

2. Antitachyarrhythmic agents are ineffective for runaway pacemaker.

3. The same therapeutic approach is indicated for other advanced malfunctions, e.g., marked slowing and/or irregular pacing (Figures 11-4 to 11-6). A new permanent pacemaker can be implanted later as an elective surgical procedure.

4. When the malfunctioning pacemaker is detected at an early stage, and when the patient is asymptomatic, the old unit can be directly replaced with a new pacemaker without first implanting a temporary device.

5. When failure of sensing and/or cardiac capture are thought to be caused by a malpositioned electrode, correction of the electrode position may be the only action necessary.

6. On the other hand, the malfunctioning pacemaker which causes a failure of sensing and/or capture should be replaced by a new unit.

7. If any factors (e.g., hyperkalemia or procainamide toxicity) responsible for producing failure of sensing and/or capture are present, they should be corrected.

8. When a broken electrode wire is responsible for the malfunction, it should be corrected accordingly.

Ventricular Fibrillation

Ventricular fibrillation may occur in any patient during insertion of a temporary pacemaker or during implantation of a permanent pacemaker. Every possible precaution should be undertaken to prevent VF.

1. If VF occurs, needless to say, immediate application of the defibrillator is mandatory.

2. Continuous intravenous infusion of lidocaine (Xylocaine; 2 to 4 mg/min) is recommended for at least 24 to 72 hr after termination of VF.

3. Some individuals may require long-term oral antiarrhythmic drug therapy [e.g., quinidine, diisopyramide phosphate (Norpace), procainamide] when frequent VPCs persist after pacing.

4. The incidence of VF is higher when a fixed-rate pacemaker is used because of the R-on-T phenomenon resulting from competition between the patient's own rhythm and the pacing-induced ventricular rhythm.

If this is the problem, in some cases a demand pacemaker should be implanted in place of a fixed-rate pacemaker.

Perforation of the Heart

Perforation of the heart may be avoided in most cases when the technical aspects for temporary as well as permanent pacing are improved. When the major complications (e.g., myocardial rupture, laceration of the cardiac valves, cardiac tamponade) occur, appropriate surgery should be performed immediately. On the other hand, minor complications (e.g., partial penetration of the catheter into the myocardium) can be corrected by repositioning the pacing electrode.

Infections

Infections related to artificial pacemaker implantation are not a frequent complication, but once present they seem to recur in some patients.

1. An infected wound requires removal of the pacing system and reimplantation elsewhere in most cases.
2. A tight wound requires revision, and it should be ascertained that the culture is negative.
3. Common organisms responsible for infections are *Staphylococcus aureus* and *Staph. epidermidis*.
4. Proper organism-sensitive antibiotics—including methicillin sodium (Staphcillin), gentamicin sulfate (Garamycin), oxacillin sodium (Prostaphlin), cephalothin sodium (Keflin), cephalexin monohydrate (Keflex), dicloxacillin sodium monohydrate (Dynapen, Pathocil, Veracillin), penicillin V potassium, streptomycin, and albamycin T (novobiocin plus tetracycline)—have been used in various combinations with varying degrees of success.
5. Unfortunately, however, antibiotic therapy alone is usually not very effective in most patients with severe infections after pacing. Thus in addition to appropriate antibiotics, radical surgery (removal of the entire infected pacemaker generator plus electrode followed by implantation of a new generator-electrode system) is almost always indicated for severe infections, particularly in patients with bacteremia and endocarditis.

Thromboembolic Phenomena

Recognition of thromboembolic phenomena, particularly pulmonary embolism and infarction, is extremely important because sudden death may occur if the problem is not diagnosed early and treated properly. Pulmonary embolism should be suspected when the patient develops unexplained dyspnea or persistent tachycardia, chest pain, or refractory heart failure. Early administration of anticoagulant therapy may prevent a lethal thromboembolic complication.

Pacemaker Sounds

Most pacemaker sounds are merely of intellectual interest and are clinically insignificant. However, perforation of the myocardium must be suspected in every patient with an artificial pacemaker in whom friction rubs are noted.

Miscellaneous Problems

Various problems related to artificial pacemakers have already been discussed in this chapter.

Artificial Pacing: Follow-up Care

12

The earliest pacemakers were implanted at thoracotomy in one of a few specialized centers, and a prolonged convalescence followed this major operative procedure. Today the majority of pacemaker leads are implanted transvenously, and the pulse generator is placed under local anesthesia. The procedure is performed in the majority of hospitals in the United States. After a day or two, the patient goes home to a new life with a pacemaker. In those short days in the hospital, healing and rehabilitation must begin simultaneously. Errors in patient care at this time may lead to troubles at a later date.

TEMPORARY PACING

Temporary transvenous pacing is nearly always instituted under fluoroscopy and monitoring in a specialized hospital unit. Often insertion is done during the daytime, and problems erupt during the night. Simple errors at the beginning may produce a catastrophe later. The principles of follow-up care after the institution of temporary pacing are similar to those which apply after the implantation of permanent pacemakers.

Care of Temporary Pacemakers

The principles governing the care of a patient with a newly implanted transvenous pacemaker are as follows:

1. A full electrocardiogram (ECG) and a chest radiograph are obtained as soon as possible after implantation for documentation and comparison.
2. The threshold is recorded and the measurement repeated daily. The dial is set to deliver 2 to 4 mA or 1 to 2 volts more than the threshold.
3. The stimulus intensity, rate, and setting of the sensitivity dial are

recorded and are regarded as physician's orders, as well-intentioned personnel otherwise might change a setting to the detriment of the clinical situation.
4. The faceplate is securely attached so that unintentional alterations do not occur.
5. Connections are checked frequently—at least once a day.
6. The date of the last battery change is written on the generator. The number of hours the generator has been in use is also recorded. Spare batteries and generators must be immediately available.
7. It is a good idea to record electrograms daily.
8. The wound is checked frequently.

Sensing Problems with Temporary Systems

If undersensing occurs, there is a danger that a pacing impulse might fall during the ventricular vulnerable phase and initiate ventricular tachyarrhythmias (VTs). Undersensing often occurs in the middle of the night, and simple measures may fail. How should one be guided?

1. The danger of VT or ventricular fibrillation (VF) is greatest in patients with acute ischemia. It is seldom of importance in any other clinical circumstance.
2. Consider whether pacing is still needed. It may be preferable to leave the pacemaker in situ but switched off. Continued monitoring is essential in case the decision is erroneous.
3. Overdrive pacing at a quite rapid rate (90 to 110 beats/min) may override the competing intrinsic ventricular focus.
4. Unipolar systems usually sense better than bipolar systems. To *unipolarize* a bipolar temporary pacing system, disconnect the pin leading to the proximal electrode and connect the positive terminal of the generator to a subcutaneous needle by means of a cable with alligator clips.
5. Intracavitary electrograms are usually better than radiographic studies for demonstrating the position of the electrode.
6. A long pause without QRS complexes or pacemaker artifacts is not pacemaker failure; it is oversensing (see below). Reducing the sensitivity or switching to an asynchronous mode is indicated in an emergency situation.
7. If all of the above-mentioned considerations fail to help, the electrode will have to be repositioned under fluoroscopic control.
8. There are some unusual cases—usually with massive myocardial infarction (MI) involving the ventricular septum—in which stable demand pacing may not be maintained.

PERMANENT PACING

Documentation of the Implant

It is essential at the outset to document the implant thoroughly. Errors and problems during follow-up may occur if the initial facts and figures are incompletely or incorrectly recorded. All data should be written in the chart at the time of implantation and should also be included in the discharge summary. The essential data to be recorded are as follows:

1. Name of the manufacturer(s), model number(s), serial number(s), and type of pulse generator and electrodes.
2. The threshold, which is defined as the lowest amount of energy at a given pulse duration that consistently paces the heart.
   a. It is incorrect to measure threshold on the way up; it must always be measured on the way down.
   b. The measurement is repeated three times and the worst measurement recorded.
   c. Threshold is measured with the stimulation pulse of the same duration as that of the pulse generator to be implanted.
   d. Threshold should be expressed in volts, although milliamperes are more commonly used.
   e. It is good practice to record a *strength-duration curve*.

Intracavitary electrograms are recorded at the same time the pacing catheter is inserted. In a temporary system they are serially recorded afterward. The following facts about electrograms should be noted:

1. They demonstrate the signal available for sensing.
2. The unipolar electrogram is more reliable than fluoroscopy for localizing the catheter.
3. They demonstrate S-T segment elevation, which indicates good contact with the endocardium; excessive wedging produces a monophasic action potential.
4. They diagnose perforation of the heart as well as fracture or short circuit of the lead, both of which are possible.

Early Postoperative Studies

It is essential to obtain a 12-lead ECG to document pacing, including capture and, if possible, sensing; a chest x-ray is also required to document the initial position of the lead. Later chest films may be compared using a superimposition technique.

Immediate Postimplant Care

1. Postimplant care must include measures to take care of surgical wounds, pain, and sleep.

2. Medications necessary for underlying cardiac disease and for any other conditions the patient may have are given.

3. It is the practice of many to use routine antibiotics, although their value in this situation has not been convincingly demonstrated. Our practice is to use a single broad spectrum antibiotic for 3 days after surgery.

4. After thoracotomy, underwater drainage and respiratory therapy are invaluable.

Cardiac Arrhythmias

1. Continuous monitoring should be used for 24 to 72 hr. This ensures that the pacemaker is functioning correctly and that any early malfunction is detected.

2. The nursing staff must be trained to recognize the interactions of an artificial pacemaker and the cardiac electrical system, as well as pacemaker-induced or related cardiac arrhythmias.

3. These include failure to capture and failure to sense, discussed below.

4. Ventricular premature contractions (VPCs) that have a configuration very similar to the paced beats may occur. These arise at the electrode-myocardial interface. They are usually benign and disappear within a day or two.

5. If necessary, VPCs may be abolished with an antiarrhythmic agent, e.g., lidocaine.

6. If VPCs persist, they may indicate that there is too much pressure on the myocardium and that perforation may follow.

Position and Activity

1. The patient should be encouraged not to lie on the right side for several days.

2. It is suggested that patients be kept on their backs for 12 hr only and then have them begin ambulation.

3. Some surgeons recommend that patients walk around with the right arm immobilized.

4. A stool softener may be used to prevent straining.

Common Early Malfunctions

The most common cause of early pacemaker malfunction (see Chapter 11) is movement of the lead or dislodgement of the catheter. The electrode may be free in the right ventricle, right atrium, or vena cava; it may lie in the coronary sinus; or it may perforate the heart. Only rarely is the generator at fault.

Failure of Cardiac Capture

Failure of cardiac capture is recognized by the discovery of a pacemaker artifact without an ensuing QRS complex that occurs at a time when the ventricles are expected to be nonrefractory. This is usually quite obvious. Confusion sometimes arises with unipolar systems that have a large pacemaker artifact. A trial capture may be especially difficult to ascertain. It may be necessary to examine the complexes in many leads to be sure. Rarely, a ventricular fusion beat causes a very small QRS complex and may be thought to be a failure of capture. Atrial capture may be difficult to detect if the P wave is swamped in the unipolar artifact.

Failure of Sensing

Failure to sense includes:

1. *Undersensing*. This is characterized by the appearance of a pacemaker artifact despite the presence of a QRS complex. It indicates that insufficient electrical signal is reaching the sensing circuit. The danger is that of stimulation within the vulnerable phase and the production of

repetitive ventricular arrhythmias or VF as a result of the R-on-T phenomenon. This is dangerous in acute ischemic conditions.

2. *Oversensing*. "Pauses without causes" suggest oversensing. The pacemaker may be sensing P waves, T waves, skeletal muscle contraction, or external electrical interference.

Perforation of the Heart

Perforation of the heart usually occurs on about the third or fourth day after implant and results in sensing or pacing failure, pericardial rub, or chest wall stimulation. Occasionally, the direction of the QRS complex in lead V_1 has changed. Normally, with right ventricular pacing there is a dominantly negative QRS complex in lead V_1. If the electrode were to migrate on to the left ventricle, a dominantly positive deflection in lead V_1 might result.

Pericardial Rub

A pericardial rub may suggest perforation or postcardiotomy syndrome.

Loss of Tissue Vitality

Infection, erosion, and dehiscence of the surgical wound may occur, resulting in a loss of tissue vitality.

Stimulation of the Diaphragm or Chest Muscles

At the time of implantation it should be demonstrated with maximum voltage that there is no skeletal muscle stimulation. Late onset diaphragmatic or intercostal pacing usually indicates partial perforation or malposition of the lead.

Pacemaker Sounds

A pacemaker sound is a sharp click that precedes the first sound and recurs 6 to 10 msec after the pacemaker artifact. It is caused by stimulation of a chest wall muscle.

Patient Participation

1. Education, like rehabilitation, should begin early.
2. The more a patient knows about his or her pacemaker, the more comfortable he or she will feel with it.
3. Education is best carried out by an enthusiastic nursing staff.
4. The patient must be given an identification card and must know the type of pacemaker implanted, the general principles of the way a pacemaker acts, and why it is needed.
5. The patient must be taught how to count his or her pulse.
6. The patient must be taught what to expect as the pacemaker functions and what to expect if it malfunctions.
7. The patient must be encouraged to return to normal activities.
8. Limitations, if any, must be spelled out.
9. The family or companions must also be included in the teaching.
10. The extremely anxious, the infirm, and the elderly are most in need of support.
11. Finally, the inpatient education program leads naturally into the follow-up system.

Artificial Pacemaker Clinics

13

For the first 15 years of clinical implantable artificial cardiac pacing, pulse generators were almost universally powered by mercury-zinc cells. The earliest units were confidently predicted to last 5 years, based on calculations of chemical energy available and current drain. It soon became clear that generators did not last 5 years; most lasted about 18 months. Indeed, some failed very early, and some failed catastrophically. The pacemaker clinic has evolved in *an attempt to predict pacemaker failure and to prolong the life of working units* which would otherwise have been replaced at arbitrary elective intervals.

In 1972 a generator using a lithium iodide battery as a power source was introduced into clinical practice. This was the first chemical power source shown to have a truly extended life. Other lithium-based chemical systems have followed. There are many lithium power sources available today, including lithium silver chromate, lithium lead iodide, lithium thionyl chloride, lithium copper sulfide, and lithium bromine systems—all with different decay and discharge characteristics. Two nuclear systems and a rechargeable system also exist.

The early, large lithium iodide cells have tended to live up to the claims of exceptional longevity and reliability. Unfortunately, the pressures of a competitive market and the desire for a cosmetic diminution in the size of the generator have led to even smaller batteries and more fanciful projections of battery life. Many have come to believe that a lithium cell (any lithium cell) would never fail. The tiniest lithium cells are failing, and probably ahead of time, perhaps because a small cell is inherently less rugged than a large one. Several lithium chemical systems have fallen into disuse today so that only lithium iodide and lithium copper sulfide are now in common usage in the United States.

Circuits have evolved also. The original circuits were discrete; and transistors, resistors, and capacitors were individually soldered and connected on a circuit board. Greater reliability has been achieved by the use of hybrid and integrated circuits in which some or all of the circuit is manufactured by machine and can be miniaturized—a "chip."

At the same time the number of companies manufacturing pacemakers has increased. The models available have multiplied to almost unmanageable levels. During the early 1960s pacing was confined to few specialized medical centers which provided careful clinical and technical follow-up. Nowadays, pacemaker implantation is being performed in a majority of hospitals and by a majority of cardiologists and cardiac surgeons in the United States as well as in many European countries. *Pacemaker clinics act as a repository of technical information* and provide a follow-up with strong medical and engineering background for patients who may have quite complex problems.

The role of the pacemaker clinic in cardiology practice is changing even more during the 1980s. Statistical results of earlier models are not applicable today, although their lessons should not be forgotten. Some of the complications that were once common may not be encountered today, e.g., ethylene oxide entrapment. Many programmers are available to change one or many functions of a generator. The clinic coordinates and regulates these actions for the greatest benefit of the patient. Pacemaker systems are continually changing, driven by medical engineering and/or marketing forces. Pacemaker clinics must evolve with them.

Background Information

1. The *necessary information for running a pacemaker clinic* is not found easily, if at all, in standard medical journals. It is available to some extent from the manufacturers. A clinic can obtain details of changes in this rapidly evolving field from the manufacturers' representatives and from the manufacturers directly. Thus the clinic acts as a repository of knowledge.

2. An *artificial pacemaker* consists of:

Pulse generator
Insulated lead
Electrode—the uninsulated part of the lead in contact with the heart
Electrode-myocardial interface

3. *Generators* may be the asynchronous or "demand" type. A demand pacemaker has two functions, i.e., to stimulate and capture the heart and to sense and respond appropriately to intrinsic electrical (QRS) signals.

4. *Pacing failure or malfunction* may occur in either or both functions and in any of the four components of the system. A unit that has been noted clinically to be functioning improperly is explanted and, on analysis, is found to be out of specification.

5. The pacemaker's *end of life* may be defined as the time when the probability of correct pacing in the near term is not clinically acceptable. Such probabilities are beginning to be known for many systems now. This definition includes important clinical considerations. Clearly,

if the patient is not dependent on his or her pacemaker, a greater leeway exists.

6. *Cumulative survival analysis*—the "actuarial method" long used to evaluate cancer therapy—allows us to calculate the time to, for example, 10% failures (90% survival), or any other figure.

7. Two other terms merit definition. Programming alters the parameters of the pacemaker noninvasively. By convention, *programmability* refers to the changes in rate and/or output. The ability to change more features is termed *multiprogrammability*. The ability to change sensitivity, output, and mode (single chamber to dual chamber) may eliminate the need for reoperation. Multiprogrammability has led the way to dual chamber pacing.

8. *Telemetry*. A special circuit in the generator can be interrogated by an external signal and can respond by broadcasting information about the battery and other functions. When the interrogating head is connected to a printer via a microcomputer, much of the information needed for the pacemaker clinic visit is readily at hand.

Detection of the Pacemaker End of Life

1. Pacemaker failure can be time-dependent (as in battery exhaustion) or random.

2. Time-dependent failures should be predictable; random, or unpredictable, failures should be detected as soon as possible.

3. In an array of mercury cells, one will fail first.

4. The circuit can be designed so that the resulting drop in voltage causes a drop in rate. The pacemaker clinic may detect this change and arrange replacement. The earliest units had no such end-of-life indicator.

5. The motor drive of conventional electrocardiographic (ECG) equipment is not always consistent from day to day and may depend on such things as fluctuations in the line voltage. It is therefore necessary to measure the generator rate with a somewhat more sophisticated instrument, the rate-interval counter. Considerable effort has been expended in following the rate of pacemakers in order to determine this small change.

6. The results of accurate measurement of pacemaker rates and intervals have been somewhat confusing and disappointing. There are several reasons for this:

1. If one cell of a battery fails in a short-circuit mode, the other cells will fail very rapidly, giving no time for a warning change of rate to be observed.
2. The components may change their values as they age, leading to changing rates. This slow drift may confuse the issue.
3. Certain circuit faults can accelerate current drain and give the impression of premature battery exhaustion. For example, when the mercury-zinc cell was improved (Mallory "certified" cells), in many models there was an increase in circuit failures for a number of reasons but the cells had good longevity.

4. The significance of a given rate change varies markedly from one manufacturer to another and from one model to another. A change of a few beats per minute after 4 to 5 months of pacing in one model may be quite acceptable, whereas in another it may indicate a serious abnormality.

7. The pacemaker clinic therefore must obtain from the manufacturers and from other pacemaker clinics as much information as possible about the expected behavior of each model.

8. Moreover, measuring pacemaker rate is only one aspect of such a patient's care. It is necessary to study the patient himself as well as all available parameters of the pacing system.

Mechanics of an Artificial Pacemaker Clinic

The necessary equipment consists of the following:

1. Oscilloscope to display the ECG
2. ECG equipment to record selected rhythm strips
3. Storage oscilloscope, enabling display of the wave form of the pacemaker artifacts, which can then be photographed with a Polaroid camera and measured for both amplitude and duration
4. Selection of magnets, ring-shaped (toroid) and horseshoe
5. Programmers and printers for all types of programmable pacemakers likely to be encountered
6. Rate-interval counter, which displays the spike-to-spike interval in milliseconds and may also automatically display the pacing rate per minute
7. Equipment with the ability to measure pulse width
8. Suitable record-keeping systems and reference materials

Procedures

The following procedures should be followed at all interviews.

1. The ECG should be observed by the physician on the oscilloscope for at least 5 min.

2. Shorter periods of observation may cause one to miss intermittent failure to capture or failure to sense. This can be done quite easily while talking to the patient and obtaining a history of recent Stokes-Adams seizures, suspicious dizzy spells, etc. *A return of symptoms needs evaluation!*

3. The *pulse generator, electrodes, and associated scars are examined for erosion, infection, adhesions, and migration.*

4. It is determined and noted if the unit is correctly *capturing and sensing*.

5. The function of the reed switch and if the patient is pacemaker-dependent are noted.

6. If the patient is in a dominant intrinsic rhythm, e.g., sinus rhythm or atrial fibrillation (AF), a *suitable magnet* is applied, which should

revert the generator to an asynchronous mode. A *magnetic interval* is then obtained and recorded. Carotid sinus massage, the Valsalva maneuver, or other vagatonic maneuvers may slow the heart sufficiently to allow the generator to take over. The *automatic interval* (the free running rate) is then obtained. Correct sensing can usually be easily inferred.

7. If the patient is in a dominant paced rhythm, one must *determine the sensing function*. Resetting and delay of the pacemaker impulse after an intrinsic beat indicates that the unit can sense that intrinsic beat. This may happen spontaneously.

8. If this does not happen, one must attempt to inhibit the generator. Several methods are available.

1. When a magnet is moved up and down over the generator with a suitable waving action, it will produce an intermittent action of the reed switch that interrupts the flow of current in a circuit; this ''break'' produces an electromotive force. The resulting voltage may be interpreted by the sensing circuit of the generator as a QRS complex and may inhibit the pacing stimuli. If this is repeated with a suitable rhythm, the generator may be inhibited for a few seconds. This is more easily done with some models than others.
2. Another method is to use an *external programmer* (in particular the Cordis Omnicor programmer), which operates by sending out powerful magnetic impulses. If the programmer is correctly positioned over the generator and the button is pressed repeatedly with a suitable rhythm, it is possible to inhibit nearly all pulse generators for a fairly prolonged period.
3. A third method is to apply *chest-wall stimulation*. Impulses are applied via suction cup electrodes to the chest wall from an external pacemaker at a rate faster than that of the implanted generator. It is usually easy to inhibit unipolar systems by this method with one electrode at the V_1 position and another at the lead V_4 position. Biopolar generators are more difficult to inhibit: Placement of the external electrodes is crucial. However, with sufficient time for exploration of the chest, it is always possible to inhibit an internal generator, provided the sensing circuit is working.

Inhibition of the pulse generator by any of these three methods simply shows that the sensing circuit is working. It does not necessarily indicate that the generator would sense a QRS complex.

9. In the majority of cases, however, an escape beat appears. With a little practice one can learn the trick of ceasing the inhibiting maneuvers in time to allow a beat to escape, followed by an impulse from the implanted generator at the correct escape interval. This would be proof that the unit can sense the patient's intrinsic beats.

10. A more prolonged application of the inhibiting maneuver would allow a succession of escape beats to appear, leading to an escape rhythm if in fact it can do so. This enables one to foretell what would happen if the pacemaker were suddenly to cease operating.

11. Some patients have a very prolonged period of asystole, and others can be shown to have a reliable escape rhythm. It should be

determined in this manner if the patient is pacemaker-dependent at each visit. In the course of time, escape impulse-forming centers may become less reliable, and patients who were formerly not dependent may become dependent.

12. The magnet should be applied at every visit. Many models will change their rate in the magnetic mode, showing the function of the reed switch. Reed switches can malfunction; e.g., they can stick open or stick closed.

13. The approximate vector of the pacing artifact in the frontal and horizontal planes can be estimated from a 12-lead ECG of paced beats. Fracture of a lead wire can lead to a change in this vector.

14. During the examination the patient is asked to lie on his left side and then on his right side. Occasionally diaphragmatic, intercostal, or pectoral muscle pacing can be provoked by this change in position. Sometimes one can cause interruption of capture, which would indicate that the electrode is not firmly attached to the right ventricle.

15. The examiner should palpate and gently move the pulse generator and the lead. If there is a fracture of the lead which is in very close opposition, or if there is a partial fracture, the "break" signals so produced may cause delay of the next pacing impulse. Pacing pauses without an apparent cause indicate oversensing.

16. The patient should be asked to press his hand into his side and so put his pectoral muscles into contraction. Quite often, especially with a unipolar system, the *myopotentials* so produced may inhibit the pacemaker. Analogous maneuvers are used when the generator is on the abdomen.

17. It is general practice to record on a 12-lead ECG at the first visit and to display on the oscilloscope the extremity leads and lead V_1 on subsequent evaluations.

1. Pacing from the right ventricular apex leads to QRS complexes that show marked left axis deviation.
2. Pacing from the middle of the interventricular septum leads to the QRS axis that is about 0 degrees in the frontal plane and suggests an inferior position or, possibly, migration of the electrode.
3. If the QRS axis is at all positive, the electrode is too close to the tricuspid valve, which may lead to inappropriate sensing of the P wave.
4. Right ventricular pacing is associated with predominantly negative QRS complexes in lead V_1.
5. Positioning the electrode through the coronary sinus into the left coronary vein leads to predominantly positive complexes in lead V_1.

18. It is usual practice to display the pacemaker artifact on the storage oscilloscope at every visit.

1. On the first visit it is photographed, and visual comparisons are made subsequently.
2. A repeat photograph is taken if there is any suspicion of a change in wave form or loss of voltage.

19. Spontaneous variations in pulse width are very rare.

1. It may have been reprogrammed or inadvertently misprogrammed.
2. Certain models are designed to show an increase in pulse width with depletion of the battery; it is then important to measure the pulse width.
3. The instrument may do this, or it may be measured directly from the display of the artifact on the storage oscilloscope.

Transtelephonic Monitoring Systems

1. Transtelephonic pacemaker monitoring can be accomplished either from a hospital base or through one of several commercial organizations.

2. In all, the patient is given a transmitter and is instructed about how to use it.

3. The patient calls the clinic at a prearranged time and transmits.

4. The information transmitted could be the free running rate, the magnet rate, the rate and pulse, the ECG, the pulse width, and the effect of the magnet.

5. In the vast majority of cases in which problem-free pacing is being experienced, this information can be simply gathered by a technician for later review by the cardiologist.

6. Certainly, this is a fine system for use with patients who live far from the medical center.

7. It has the added advantage that a patient can call at unscheduled times if he thinks something is wrong with his pacemaker.

8. It does not allow the extended studies described above but can be a very useful supplement to a standard clinic.

9. It is by no means a substitute for personal medical care.

Computers

In a large, busy medical institution, it may be impossible to keep track of the various kinds of pacemaker employed. Computerization can thus be very useful. For example, should a patient appear in the emergency room at night, a well-designed system can quickly retrieve the relevant pacemaker data.

Explanted Units

It is the responsibility of the pacemaker clinic to set up a system for checking all explanted units. Some clinics prefer to have their own engineering teams analyze the units, whereas others prefer to return them to the manufacturer for possible credit and analysis (which may or may not be very thorough). Every clinic, hospital, or large medical group should have their own indications for generator replacement and should have their own statistics.

Patient Participation

1. Patients should be taught to count their own pulse for a full minute every day and record it.

2. The generator can be checked quite simply when one holds a transistor radio, tuned between stations, over it. A characteristic click can be heard as the generator fires.

3. The instruction can be reinforced, and the significance of any variation can be discussed at the time of each clinic visit. Many patients have fears and misconceptions about artificial pacemakers (as do many physicians). A kind and intelligent nurse can be an asset to the pacemaker clinic.

4. Patients may fail to keep appointments for trivial or serious reasons. ''No shows'' should be telephoned by clinic personnel as soon as possible to determine the reason for the absence.

5. It is important to maintain close relations with the patient's own physician, but the pacemaker clinic personnel should not usurp the physician's function. The clinic's function is quite distinct from that of the physician.

Frequency of Visits and Calls

1. It has been generally accepted that surveillance (by personal clinic visits and/or telephone) should be less frequent in the first year and more frequent later on, when a greater probability of pacemaker failure is anticipated.

2. Various schedules are available. A typical one might provide for calls every 3 months during the first year and then once or twice a week after 1 year. This would make sense if the predominant mode of pacemaker failure were time-dependent, but the lifetime of a lithium, nuclear, or modern rechargeable generator is not clearly known. Circuit failures tend to be randomly distributed and not to be time-dependent.

3. The most common causes of early pacemaker problems are lead displacement, perforation, and ''exit block.'' Many of these problems are related to less than perfect implantation techniques.

4. Bearing this in mind, it seems wise for patients to be seen frequently during the first few months.

5. If the patients are doing well, they could be put onto a 3- or 4-month schedule for a fairly prolonged period, during which time they would be checking their own pacemakers.

6. When the expected life of their pacemaker is known more accurately, the patients could be seen more and more frequently as the end of that lifetime is approached. This will have to be judged with great care, as no prognostications can be confidently made.

Educational Value

Those who learn most from a pacemaker clinic are the individuals who run it and work in it. A good clinic may be able to detect faults in pacemaker models that the manufacturer has not recognized. The clinic can monitor the group's own performance and identify those physicians who have a high rate of complications. Moreover, the medical and engineering teams learn about each other's discipline, and they certainly learn a lot about patients.

Suggested Reading

Braunwald, E. 1980. Heart Diseases: A Textbook of Cardiovascular Medicine, Saunders, Philadelphia.

Chung, E. K. 1976. Non-Invasive Cardiac Diagnosis, Lea & Febiger, Philadelphia.

Chung, E. K. 1979. Ambulatory Electrocardiography: Holter Monitor Electrocardiography, Springer-Verlag, New York.

Chung, E. K. 1980. Cardiac Emergency Care, 2nd Ed. Lea & Febiger, Philadelphia.

Chung, E. K. 1980. Electrocardiography: Practical Applications with Vectorial Principles, 2nd Ed. Harper/Lippincott, Philadelphia.

Chung, E. K. 1982. Heart Attack, Appleton-Century-Crofts, Norwalk, Conn.

Chung, E. K. 1982. One Heart, One Life: A Healthy Heart Handbook, Prentice-Hall, Englewood Cliffs, N.J.

Chung, E. K. 1983. Principles of Cardiac Arrhythmias, 3rd Ed. Williams & Wilkins, Baltimore.

Chung, E. K. 1983. Quick Reference To Cardiovascular Diseases, 2nd Ed. Harper/Lippincott, Philadelphia.

Chung, E. K., and Chung, L. S. 1983. Introduction To Clinical Cardiology, Karger, New York.

Furman, S., and Escher, D. J. W. 1975. Modern Cardiac Pacing: A Clinical Overview, Charles Press, Bowie, MD.

Hurst, J. W., Logue, R. B., Rackley, C. E., et al. 1976. The Heart, 5th Ed. McGraw-Hill, New York.

Lüderitz, B. 1976. Cardiac Pacing, Springer-Verlag, New York.

Schaldach, M., and Furman, S. 1975. Advances In Pacemaker Technology, Springer-Verlag, New York.

Thalen, H. J. Th., and Meere, C. 1979. Fundamentals of Cardiac Pacing, Martinus Nijhoff, The Hague.

Glossary of Abbreviations

AF Atrial fibrillation
APC Atrial premature contraction
A-V Atrioventricular
BBBB Bilateral bundle branch block
BFB Bifascicular block
BP Blood pressure
BTS Bradytachyarrhythmia syndrome
CAD Coronary artery disease
CHF Congestive heart failure
CPR Cardiopulmonary resuscitation
CSS Carotid sinus stimulation
DC shock Direct current shock
DI Digitalis intoxication
ECG Electrocardiogram
LBBB Left bundle branch block
MI Myocardial infarction
MVPS Mitral valve prolapse syndrome
PAT Paroxysmal atrial tachycardia
RBBB Right bundle branch block
RHD Rheumatic heart disease
SSS Sick sinus syndrome
TFB Trifascicular block
VF Ventricular fibrillation
VPC Ventricular premature contraction
VT Ventricular tachycardia
WPW syndrome Wolff-Parkinson-White syndrome

Artificial Pacing Inter-Society Commission for Heart Diseases (ICHD) Resource Code

Three-Letter Code

First letter—chamber paced
- A = atrium
- V = ventricle
- D = double chamber

Second letter—chamber sensed
- A = atrium
- V = ventricle
- D = double chamber
- O = none

Third letter—mode of response
- T = triggered
- I = inhibited
- D = dual (triggered and inhibited)
- O = not applicable

Five-Letter Code

First three letters—as with three letter code

Fourth letter—programmability
- P = programmable for rate and/or output
- M = multiprogrammable
- O = nonprogrammable

Fifth letter—type of response selected to treat a tachyarrhythmia
- B = bursts (groups of 3-10 beats at a rapid rate)
- N = normal (normal pacer rate to cause slow-rate blocking competition)
- S = scanning (scanning of rhythm with insertion of one blocking beat at correct time)
- E = external pulse generator (radiofrequency initiated blocking burst from external transmitter)

Examples of Pacemaker Codes

1. Asynchronous	
Atrial pacing, no sensing	AOO
Ventricular pacing, no sensing	VOO
Atrioventricular pacing, no sensing (AV sequential)	DOO
2. Triggered	
Atrial pacing and atrial sensing, triggered mode	AAT
Ventricular pacing and ventricular sensing, triggered mode (ventricular synchronous)	VVT
Ventricular pacing and atrial sensing, triggered mode (atrial synchronous)	VAT
3. Inhibited	
Atrial pacing and atrial sensing, inhibited mode	AAI
Ventricular pacing and ventricular sensing, inhibited mode (ventricular inhibited)	VVI
Atrioventricular pacing and ventricular sensing, inhibited mode (bifocal of AV sequential demand)	DVI

4. Combined
   a. Ventricular pacing and atrial sensing (VAT) — VDD
      Ventricular sensing and ventricular inhibition (VVI)
      (VAT with sensing and inhibiting ventricular output if VPCs occur)
   b. Ventricular pacing and atrial sensing (VAT) — DDD
      AV-sequential (DVI)
      (VAT becoming DVI if marked sinus bradycardia occurs)
   c. Ventricular pacing and sensing, inhibited (VVI) plus ventricular triggered (VVT)
      Atrial pacing and sensing, inhibited (AAI) plus atrial triggered (AAT)
      (VVI or AAI capable of sensing and responding to tachycardia with a short blocking burst of programmed tachycardial pacing)
5. Paired and coupled pacing
   Paired pacing — AOO or VOO
   Coupled pacing — AAT or VVT

Index

Topics and page numbers in boldface indicate areas of major discussion